Law and Ethics in Intensive Care

Law and Ethics in Intensive Care

Second edition

Edited by

Christopher Danbury

Consultant in Intensive Care Medicine,
Royal Berkshire Hospital, Reading, UK

Christopher Newdick

Professor of Health Law,
University of Reading, Reading, UK

Alex Ruck Keene

Barrister, 39 Essex Chambers;
Visiting Lecturer and Wellcome Research Fellow,
King's College London, London, UK

Carl Waldmann

Consultant in Anaesthetics and Intensive Care Medicine,
Royal Berkshire Hospital, Reading, UK

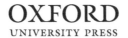

OXFORD
UNIVERSITY PRESS

OXFORD

UNIVERSITY PRESS

Great Clarendon Street, Oxford, OX2 6DP,
United Kingdom

Oxford University Press is a department of the University of Oxford.
It furthers the University's objective of excellence in research, scholarship,
and education by publishing worldwide. Oxford is a registered trade mark of
Oxford University Press in the UK and in certain other countries

First Edition published in 2010
Second Edition published in 2020

Impression: 1

Published in the United States of America by Oxford University Press
198 Madison Avenue, New York, NY 10016, United States of America

British Library Cataloguing in Publication Data

Data available

Library of Congress Control Number: 2020942396

ISBN 978-0-19-881716-1

Printed in Great Britain by
Ashford Colour Press Ltd, Gosport, Hampshire

Foreword

Thirty years ago, when medical law as we now understand it was in its infancy in this country, reported cases were few and textbooks and monographs even fewer. Today, our shelves groan under the weight of a seemingly ceaseless flow of new cases and new books.

Why is this book, whose second edition is very welcome, so important and so valuable?

First, it deals with a centrally important topic—intensive care—which, as the editors remark, presents in one medical discipline many of the most intractable problems in health law. More than many medical matters, and as this book so pervasively brings out, intensive care engages, most acutely, ethics as much as medicine and the law. And, as the editors justly observe, it is an area of medical practice where the law has not always played as helpful a part as one would hope. As they comment, at times the courts appear to place impossible demands upon clinicians in the intensive care unit.

Second, the book is multi-disciplinary, with a distinguished list of contributors from the worlds of both medicine and the law. Their core ambition is to encourage law and the realities of clinical practice to march hand in hand. That must be right, for, without debating where the balance of decision-making responsibility and power ultimately lies—a crucial question on which a number of contributors offer very important insights—, it must surely be the case that the law, medicine, and ethics march hand in hand: standing together in unison, each contributing to an outcome that is informed by a profound awareness of, and empathetic understanding for, the realities of the human condition and the dignity of the patient, and also—dare one say it—informed by a robust common sense.

Third, the book is engagingly written in a most accessible style, while never sacrificing a careful and rigorous analysis where descriptions of the clinical realities are inter-weaved with illuminating discussions of the leading cases. And, unlike too many such books, it can be read from cover to cover with pleasure as well as profit.

Medical law may have been with us for only 30 years—although, as one contributor points out, death has been part of the human condition for 200,000 years and the subject of medical study for some three centuries—but science and medical science march on, as do social and societal attitudes. Who would have thought 30 years ago that a book such as this would have to include a chapter entitled 'Social Media in Intensive Care'?

The relentless onward march of science, medicine, and law will inevitably require, and probably sooner rather than later, a third edition, but in the meantime we are indebted to the editors and their contributors for providing us with such excellent fare.

Sir James Munby, 27 July 2019
Lately President of the Family Division of the
High Court and President of the Court of Protection.

Preface to the Second Edition

The first edition of this book was published in 2010. Since then many things have changed in the worlds of medicine and the law. First, our co-editor, Dr Andrew Lawson, was diagnosed with mesothelioma. He rapidly became an expert on the disease, travelling the world for the most effective treatments. Sadly, he died after a brave and long fight. He managed to live with the illness for six years after diagnosis in which time he gave his family, friends, and colleagues the benefit of his love, wit, wisdom, and constant sense of fun. He survived long enough for one of his insurance companies to doubt the accuracy of his initial diagnosis, something that amused him enormously. It was not until very close to the end that he had to concede in his fight against this awful disease. He is a great loss and we dedicate this book to the indelible memory of his energy, his infectious good humour, and his drive to contribute to the good of intensive care medicine.

Joining our team of editors is Alex Ruck Keene. Alex is a Wellcome Research Fellow and Visiting Lecturer at King's College London; a Visiting Senior Lecturer at the Institute of Psychiatry, Psychology and Neuroscience, King's College London; and a Research Affiliate at the Essex Autonomy Project, University of Essex. He spent 2016 on secondment to the Law Commission as a consultant to their Mental Capacity and Deprivation of Liberty project and throughout 2018 was legal adviser to the Independent Review of the Mental Health Act 1983. He is a very welcome addition.

For doctors doing an intensive care ward round, ethical and legal dilemmas are associated with almost every patient, yet it is only recently that these issues have arisen in the literature and in litigation. Some, such as deprivation of liberty, looked destined to complicate every intensive care admission, at least in England and Wales, with the potential to divert time and staff away from patient care, but thankfully this threat has now subsided. Twelve years after the Mental Capacity Act 2005 came into force in England and Wales, the courts have had plenty of time to develop and refine the meaning both of capacity and best interests towards an ever more intense focus on the individual patient. At times, the courts appear to place impossible demands on clinicians in the intensive care unit, and a core interest of the co-editors of this work is to encourage law and the realities of clinical practice to march hand in hand.

Consternation has also arisen around the area of withdrawal of organ support. Several high-profile disputes have arisen where one sympathizes with all the parties involved: patients, their relatives, and clinical staff. In addition to the legal and ethical complexities these cases provoke, the contributors to this volume also raise concern for the personal cost to those involved. Mediation may offer a more sensitive and satisfactory means of responding. When mediation can develop acceptable solutions, relatives and clinicians will be spared both the stresses of litigation and, perhaps, the challenge of having to continue to cooperate closely together after the case has ended.

Intensive care presents in one medical discipline many of the most intractable problems in health law. How should the law of informed consent work when, by definition, most patients cannot express their wishes and doctors often find it difficult to predict which interventions will be appropriate, over what period of time, or how individuals will respond? The position may be still more fraught in respect of babies and children, especially when differences of opinion arise as to the best course of action. When matters cannot be resolved by agreement, cases attract public attention. Who is best placed to determine their best interests: patients, parents, doctors, or the courts—and how can mediation help?

At the centre is always the patient, and their voice must have the greatest influence. However, as Donne said, 'No man is an island,' and so other players should also be heard. Reflecting these concerns, this book is divided into three parts. Part A is concerned with the challenges involved in hearing the patient's voice. Dominic Bell illuminates the challenges presented by the increasingly patient-centred model of informed consent and considers how best to respond to the uncertainties endemic to intensive care practice. Alex Ruck Keene and Zoë Fritz raise the difficult issues encountered when patients refuse or demand medical care. Hazel Biggs discusses 'Do not attempt resuscitation' orders, the challenge of consistency of practice, and the need to communicate these sensitive matters candidly to patients themselves.

Part B turns the focus towards the voice of others intimately concerned with patients' welfare, especially doctors, parents, and relatives. Babies and young children stir our deepest emotions, never more so than when they are in poor health in intensive care, and Thérèse Callus considers the role of parents in balancing and deciding best interests. Who should have the final word in these cases and according to which test? Daniele Bryden deals with patients who lack capacity and the range of 'best interest' options available under the Mental Capacity Act 2005. Chris Newdick and Chris Danbury assess the notion of 'futility' in intensive care, the extraordinary difficulties that surround the notion and role of mediation to encourage trust and confidence. Dale Gardiner and Andrew McGee consider the many modern controversies that continue to confront doctors in the diagnosis of death, be they philosophical, clinical, legal, or religious.

Part C addresses the various external influences that bear on these questions. Louise Austin and John Coggon assess the legal relevance of the wider, altruistic concerns of intensive care patients themselves with the best interests of others who may benefit from a donation of their organs after they die. Neil Soni, the late Andrew Lawson, and Carl Waldmann raise the various conflicts of interest that arise from the close relationship that has developed between commerce and healthcare, and the contribution of the Academy of Medical Royal Colleges. Finally, Rosaleen Baruah is concerned with the rise of the influence of social media on public perceptions and the new pressures this brings to the intensive care ward.

We emphasize the idea of 'listening' because the collective experience of practitioners in this field is of the value of candid communication and the unfortunate tensions that will arise when relations break down. We cannot cover every legal and ethical issue in intensive care, but we have endeavoured to discuss those we consider most topical and challenging.

CD, CN, ARK, CW

Preface to the First Edition

The practice of intensive care is being transformed. Demographic changes mean that more of us live to a good age and will require intensive care later in our lives. Pharmaceutical and medical technologies have introduced a range of treatments, which for many are life-saving, but for others have less significant impact and leave them in a fragile and uncertain condition. Patients and their relatives have seen their rights in this area transformed, so that the old paternalistic approaches of the past have been replaced with a duty to be open, to discuss, and to negotiate. And, of course, there is the pressure of NHS governance and the need to manage the risk of litigation if things go wrong.

The great American jurist, Charles Warren, once said that the law floats on a sea of ethics. Modern critical care medicine too provokes multiple ethical and legal problems, which make it even more difficult to know who and when to admit to intensive care, at what stage should invasive management be withdrawn, and who should decide. These profound dilemmas, made more complicated in a setting of scarce resources, mandate an understanding of relevant contemporary laws and the ethical principles that underpin our actions. This collection of articles on ethical and legal aspects of intensive care medicine is published at a crucial time both in the evolution of critical care medicine but also with respect to the way society is responding to health care challenges.

The book addresses a variety of ethical controversies in the United Kingdom relevant to our speciality. Although there [is] inevitable overlap, we have divided the book into a series of sections as follows: Part A addresses issues of competency and autonomy and includes chapters by Bell on 'Consent for Intensive Care—Public and Political Expectations vs. Conceptual and Practical Hurdles', Bryden on 'Adults Who Lack Capacity to Consent', and Newdick and Danbury on 'the Best Interests of Babies and Children'. Part B focuses on issues between doctor and patient, with chapters by McLean and Morgan on 'Taking it or Leaving It: Demanding and Refusing Treatment in Intensive Care', Biggs on 'Dying to Know: Legal and Ethical Issues Surrounding Death and Do Not Resuscitate Orders', Lawson on 'Diagnosing Death', and Woodcock on 'Research in Intensive Care'. Finally, Part C considers the challenges of managing the intensive care unit, with contributions from Pittaway and Peacock on 'NHS Governance of Critical Care', Newdick and Danbury on 'Reverse Triage? Managing Scarce Resources', Coggon on 'Doing What's Best: Organ Donation and Intensive Care', and Waldmann, Soni, and Lawson on 'Conflicts of Interest'.

Although not comprehensive, we have developed key issues of interests to intensivists, and the chapter authors have been selected for their reputation and passion for the subject. We hope that there is something useful for everybody in this book.

CD, CN, AL, CW

Contents

PART C. EXTERNAL INFLUENCES

Contributors to the First Edition

Dr Dominic Bell
Consultant in Intensive Care/Anaesthesia,
The General Infirmary at Leeds,
UK

Professor Hazel Biggs
Professor of Medical Law,
School of Law,
University of Southampton,
UK

Dr Margaret Branthwaite
Retired Barrister,
Formerly Consultant in Anaesthesia,
Intensive Care and Respiratory Medicine,
Royal Brompton Hospital,
UK

Dr Daniele C. Bryden
Consultant in Intensive Care Medicine and
Anaesthesia,
Sheffield Teaching Hospitals,
NHS Trust,
UK

Dr John Coggon
British Academy Postdoctoral Fellow
School of Law,
University of Manchester,
UK

Dr Christopher Danbury
Consultant in Intensive Care Medicine and
Anaesthetics,
Royal Berkshire Hospital,
UK

Dr Andrew Lawson
Honorary Senior Lecturer,
Medical Ethics, Imperial College
Post Graduate Student,
Worcester College, Oxford,
UK

Professor S. A. M. McLean
International Bar Association,
Chair of Law and Ethics in Medicine,
School of Law,
University of Glasgow,
UK

Dr Derek Morgan
Professor of Medical Law and
Jurisprudence,
School of Law,
University of Sheffield,
UK

Professor Christopher Newdick
School of Law,
The University of Reading,
UK

Nicholas A. Peacock
Barrister,
Hailsham Chambers,
UK

David Pittaway QC
Barrister,
Hailsham Chambers,
UK

Dr Neil Soni
Consultant in Intensive Care and
Anaesthetics,
Chelsea and Westminster,
Hospital,
UK

Dr Carl Waldmann
Consultant Intensive Care and
Anaesthesia,
Royal Berkshire Hospital,
UK

Dr Thomas E. Woodcock
Consultant in Intensive Care and
Anaesthetics,
Southampton University,
NHS Trust,
UK

Contributors to the Second Edition

Louise Austin, Lecturer in Law, Cardiff University, Cardiff, UK

Rosaleen Baruah, Consultant in Intensive Care Medicine, Western General Hospital, Edinburgh, Scotland, UK

Dominic Bell, Consultant in Intensive Care Medicine, Leeds Hospital NHS Trust, Leeds, UK

Hazel Biggs, Professor of Healthcare Law and Bioethics, University of Southampton Law School, and Health Ethics and Law (HEAL), University of Southampton, Southampton, UK

Daniele Bryden, Consultant in Intensive Care Medicine and Anaesthesia, Sheffield Teaching Hospitals NHS Foundation Trust; Honorary Senior Lecturer, University of Sheffield, Sheffield, UK

Thérèse Callus, Professor of Law, School of Law, University of Reading, Reading, UK

John Coggon, Professor of Law, Centre for Health, Law, and Society, University of Bristol Law School, UK

Christopher Danbury, Consultant in Intensive Care Medicine, Royal Berkshire Hospital, Reading, UK

Zoë Fritz, Consultant in Acute Medicine, Cambridge University Hospitals, and Wellcome Fellow in Society and Ethics, THIS (The Healthcare Improvement Studies Institute), University of Cambridge, UK

Dale Gardiner, Consultant in Intensive Care Medicine, Nottingham University Hospitals NHS Trust; National Clinical Lead for Organ Donation, NHS Blood and Transplant, Bristol, UK

Alex Ruck Keene, Barrister, 39 Essex Chambers; Visiting Lecturer and Wellcome Research Fellow, King's College London, London, UK

The late **Andrew Lawson**, Former Honorary Senior Lecturer, Medical Ethics, Imperial College, and Former Post Graduate Student, Worcester College, Oxford, UK

Andrew McGee, Associate Professor, Australian Centre for Health Law Research, Faculty of Law, Queensland University of Technology, Brisbane, Queensland, Australia

Christopher Newdick, Professor of Health Law, University of Reading, Reading, UK

Neil Soni, Formerly Consultant in Anaesthesia and Intensive Care Medicine, Chelsea and Westminster Hospital, London, UK

Carl Waldmann, Consultant in Anaesthetics and Intensive Care Medicine, Royal Berkshire Hospital, Reading, UK

PART A

LISTENING TO PATIENTS

1

Consent for Intensive Care

Public and Political Expectations vs. Conceptual and Practical Hurdles

Dominic Bell

Introduction

A decade ago, in the first iteration of this chapter, the barriers to meeting contemporary expectations on consent were explored, principally the difficulties in defining intensive care, providing a prognosis not only on survival but on the quality of life in the event of survival, and accommodating individual preferences and changing values and beliefs in response to provision of care. These core issues remain unresolved as will be expanded on within the chapter, but this should not be interpreted as consent remaining a static topic over this interval. The legal case of *Montgomery v Lanarkshire Health Board*[1] has not only shifted provision of information firmly away from medical discretion and implied that this principle has historically been applicable, but is also clearly relevant to everyday intensive care decision making with patients and their relatives by specifying that treatment options should not be withheld from the patient to consider purely on the basis that the practitioner does not consider a certain approach appropriate. The concern that, for a significant proportion of patients, intensive care constitutes a 'deprivation of liberty' when evaluated against the principles of the Mental Capacity Act 2005, thereby requiring the authorization or 'proxy consent' of independent statutory bodies, has been a significant distraction for practitioners over the past ten years as analysed within subsequent chapters. The past decade also witnessed a large-scale media campaign and public backlash against the Liverpool Care Pathway, particularly once it was realized that healthcare providers were reimbursed for compliance under Commissioning for Quality and Innovation (CQUIN) arrangements,[2] thus bringing under the spotlight end-of-life care, medical paternalism and both provision of information and the exploration of individual values and beliefs when seeking consent or assent in this field of practice. There are warnings in any analysis of these events when assessing the rapidly changing approach to organ donation over the past ten years, the fundamental question remaining as to what can legitimately be assumed as accommodated within 'consent' expressed via registration as an organ donor or on an individual's behalf by the next of kin. It can be argued that the very use of trained facilitators in the form of specialist nurses for organ donation with progressive exclusion of clinical requesting runs contrary to the fundamental principles of consent, and the push towards withdrawal of support in the anaesthetic room and on the operating theatre table as objectives for optimal organ retrieval, further emphasizes this point. More recent organ donation initiatives in the form of active intervention for 'devastating brain injury' also demonstrate challenges to the concept of consent, and it is apparent therefore that professional bodies as well as individual clinicians will continue to tread a fine line if a public backlash is to be avoided, particularly in the aftermath of *Montgomery*. As Parliament moves ever closer to enacting 'presumed consent', a concept totally at odds with fundamental principles of consent, it is foreseeable that these intrinsic contradictions and shortfalls will be highlighted. A further interesting development over this time frame is the devolution of authority for the withdrawal of nutrition and hydration from individuals in a chronic prolonged disorder of consciousness to the healthcare team in conjunction with the next of kin, a significant shift from the previous model whereby the Court of Protection had responsibility for determining the lawfulness or otherwise of what was proposed. It remains to be seen whether the removal of an independent tier of scrutiny for such decisions will engender a return to medical paternalism with respect to joint decision making on these matters of societal significance, and ultimately trigger public concern as to the lack of accountability of the profession. All these issues are therefore playing out as the backdrop to everyday decision making in critical care in which it would be predictably difficult to evidence compliance with the standards of consent that have been adopted by the majority of mainstream specialties. The goal of this chapter is to analyse the nature and history of both intensive care and consent before assessing whether contemporary standards for informed consent are achievable for intensive care, while highlighting the areas where the specialty could reasonably demonstrate understanding of, and compliance with, the underlying principles.

Background

Intensive care is a complex subject, predictably intangible and difficult to understand for the general public, or indeed for many other medical disciplines. The simple origins of this specialty within ventilatory support for paralysis, or as a continuation of resuscitation or peri-operative care, have served to define our practice as an extension of treatment initiated by others, rather than a discrete intervention appropriate for proactive patient choice. The overall historical style of mainly non-standardized care, delivered by part-time practitioners, limited post-discharge treatment or audit of outcomes, and patient ownership resting with the parent specialty, served to maintain this position, with little public scrutiny of process.

Recent years have, however, seen independent specialty status, formalized training and accreditation, and an increasingly standardized process of care as the evidence base for effective treatments expands with robust research and consensus guidelines. The philosophy of intensive care has also changed over this time frame, with greater emphasis on early identification of the at-risk patient within the broader hospital, timely implementation of treatments to modify critical illness, and the accompanying opportunity for proactive engagement with patient and next of kin, prior to the point of decompensation. With a more defined treatment strategy, greater knowledge of outcomes, and the opportunity for earlier discussion with the patient, it could reasonably be expected that intensive care parallels all other medical interventions, with informed consent directing the approach.

Consent to medical treatment is historically founded in common law as an essential process to distinguish surgical activity from actionable assault, but the concept has become progressively refined to represent the profession's ethical rather than strictly legal duty to respect the autonomy, or right to self-determination, of the patient. This transition from medical paternalism has paralleled the universal rise of broader human rights, but has been particularly fuelled within the UK by scandals involving the withholding of information from patients on the outcomes from cardiac surgery[3] and post-mortem procedure.[4] New legislation such as the Human Tissue Act 2004[5] was borne out of the subsequent public and political dissatisfaction, placing great emphasis on the comprehensiveness of information and full understanding of what is involved. The standard now demanded by the courts is not what the healthcare professional believes is reasonable to disclose, or their perspective on the significance of any risk materializing, but what the individual patient may interpret as significant,[6] a principle endorsed in *Montgomery*. These standards are further emphasized within recommendations from defence societies, government, and professional bodies,[7, 8] raising the argument that the law is simply catching up with and emphasizing long-established ethical principles.

While the concept of 'informed consent' has never been formally enshrined in statute within the UK therefore, there is an expectation that information will be provided in an understandable format on what is proposed and the associated risks and benefits, with a similar level of detail on alternatives, including doing nothing. There should be time enough for the patient to reflect on what is suggested, with the opportunity for further questions, and freedom from any pressure or coercion to comply with the practitioner's favoured strategy. Consent, furthermore, should be a dynamic process with constant re-evaluation of the above issues, rather than a presumption of ongoing consent simply based on continuing compliance.

A major barrier to conformity with these principles is that significant numbers of intensive care patients have already lost capacity, a fundamental prerequisite for consent, at the point of presentation and never regain this during the length of their critical illness. There are, however, opportunities for early proactive engagement in those patients with chronic disease liable to presentation with life-threatening deterioration or complications, in other patients early on in the admission process when progressive deterioration is predictable, and particularly in those patients about to undergo major surgery with a foreseeable requirement for post-operative intensive care.

It should also be noted that even for those patients whose capacity has been compromised by illness or medication, but where subsequent healthcare choices have to be undertaken, attempts should be made to promote capacity and autonomous decision making. This obligation is unequivocally spelt out within the Mental Capacity Act 2005,[9] which further emphasizes how lack of capacity is limited to a specific decision at a specific point in time, rather than a continuing feature that would prevent any consideration of choice on any subject at any time. Even with severe brain injury or dysfunction, such as dementia, the default position should be that healthcare professionals seek to determine capacity for decision making and promote this whenever possible.

Given the above-defined recommendations from the relevant authorities, the emphasis is therefore on seeking fully informed consent for all aspects of intensive care provision, mirroring every other healthcare intervention. While this approach would meet those legal requirements, the feasibility of such an undertaking has to be assessed in the first instance, and the more fundamental question of whether patients wish for such a system in relation to critical illness and end-of-life care, or prefer a style based more on 'benign paternalism', needs to be secondarily considered.

Feasibility of informed consent within critical care

In addressing the first of these challenges, the feasibility of informed consent for intensive care revolves around a series of questions.

1. Can the basic process of care be defined, and further refined for specific categories of illness?
2. How are outcomes defined and calculated?
   a. survival of critical illness
   b. survival to leave hospital
   c. longer-term survival
   d. dependence on medical intervention throughout these stages
   e. survival versus health status
   f. quality of life throughout these stages.
3. How does age, background comorbidity, and triggering pathology influence the above issues?
4. Can understanding be achieved of the ancillary facets of intensive care, such as dependency, loss of privacy, threat to personal dignity, compromised capacity, or the mental and physical effort of weaning and rehabilitation?
5. Can there be rational judgment on when the potentially temporary burdens of living during critical illness outweigh the prospects of longer-term recovery, and when this should therefore limit further life-sustaining medical treatment?
6. What degrees of certainty would an individual patient want within each of these domains to facilitate an informed decision?

This series of questions not unreasonably generates reservations as to whether it is possible to specify the clinical course of the patient along the intensive care pathway and set out the components of care that the patient might wish to partake of or decline at different stages of that pathway, and whether it is possible to carry out this exercise without compromising the normal process of coordinated care. An obvious unwanted consequence for all involved, of any attempt to comprehensively define the clinical pathway, would be the potential future restriction on a flexible approach to care depending on the patient's response to primary treatments, which is in essence the philosophy of intensive care.

The relatively recent and ultimately simplistic attempts to engage patients on proactive decision making on resuscitation[10] is illustrative of this problem—namely, that a complex decision with significant ramifications cannot and should not be reduced to a simple and rigid 'yes' or 'no'. Resuscitation manoeuvres should also be placed in the context of earlier life-sustaining medical treatment on which the patient should definitely have an opinion, because this is likely to be determinative on both the incidence of a cardiac arrest and the likely outcome.

These identified questions and further hurdles will be addressed below.

Can the process of intensive care be defined?

Intensive care is less a specific treatment for a defined pathology and more a complex amalgam of multi-system support, the need for which has been dictated by decompensation of the patient. This in turn may be due to the magnitude of the triggering pathology in a previously healthy individual, such as polytrauma or meningococcal septicaemia, may reflect underlying comorbidity such as respiratory or immune disease, or be attributable to some combination of these factors such as major surgery in the presence of established cardio-respiratory pathology. Optimization of the patient in these circumstances requires treatments, such as sedation, that have no therapeutic value other than facilitating necessary interventions, alongside invasive monitoring and multiple radiological and laboratory investigations. In many cases, intensive care is less of a treatment and more of an assessment of a patient's physiological reserve for withstanding medical or surgical illness by ongoing evaluation of their response to the various support strategies.

This difficulty in defining the principles of intensive care is amplified by the range of approaches between, and even within, units on virtually every aspect of management from choice of monitoring modality to criteria for referring for or prescribing super-tertiary treatments such as extracorporeal membrane oxygenation. The evidence base over the past decade has, however, evolved to either eliminate or significantly reduce some historical variation between units on interventions such as activated protein C, nitric oxide, and high-frequency oscillation as well as more mundane elements such as synthetic colloids. There is also international convergence and an increasing adoption of a standardized approach for certain reproducible conditions as exemplified by the Surviving Sepsis Campaign[11] or with respect to transfusion thresholds,[12] but the cyclically changing approach to induced hypothermia after cardiac arrest and brain injury demonstrates the difficulties in deriving consistency for many everyday conditions. Even basic questions, such as the optimal timing for a tracheostomy, remain unanswered, despite extensive national research on such topics,[13] and, although there will inevitably be a contribution to variation because of the intrinsic differences between individual patients, this observation alone demonstrates the limitations in applying broader outcome figures to individual patients for the purposes of consent.

The overall package of intensive care becomes even harder to define for the consent process when considering the multidisciplinary input into direct delivery of care, involving medical, nursing, and physiotherapy staff, all with independent codes of practice and different implications in relation to consent. While the medical components of care have been discussed above, nursing interventions cover diverse aspects relevant to privacy, independence, and dignity, such as personal hygiene and bowel care, while physiotherapy may involve encouragement of the patient in activities for which there is little enthusiasm or even absolute resistance, such as passive stretching, mobilization, and spontaneous ventilatory effort independent of mechanical support.

If, therefore, intensive care cannot be readily defined as a medical treatment, because of fundamental conceptual aspects coupled with significant variation in the approach to critical illness, and management involves a range of healthcare professionals each with a different impact on a patient's autonomy and personal integrity, the starting requirement for consent, in which the proposed treatment is described, is rendered problematical.

Can the indications for intensive care be defined?

Although intensive care is routinely perceived by the lay public as synonymous with being on a 'life-support machine', it is apparent that there is a spectrum of indications for ICU admission from the planned slow emergence from anaesthesia after major surgery to the continuation of the resuscitation process after decompensation of the patient following trauma, medical illness, or surgery. When one considers, furthermore, that critical care should be as much a pre-emptive process as reactive rescue care, patients at a low level of illness severity and the probability of not needing an escalation of support may be moved into such an environment for a higher intensity of monitoring associated with just basic aspects of care. By definition, this process needs to be flexible and responsive, and is often based on the subjective opinion of an experienced clinician as much as objective measures of physiological derangement such as Modified Early Warning Scores (MEWS),[14] creating difficulty with translation into a specific template for the purposes of consent.

Furthermore, intensive care is a process of patient management rather than a geographical location, and logistical issues may at times dictate that the critically ill patient requiring multi-system support will have this delivered in a non-designated area, and at times the patient with a lower severity of illness may be monitored in an ICU bed in the absence of step-down availability. It would be too simplistic, therefore, and inappropriately restrictive of future choice to have absolute restrictions on admission to intensive care, as a geographical resource, as a component of proactive consent.

Can the prognosis from, and the goals of, intensive care be defined?

When considering the spectrum of indications for admission to intensive care as set out above, it would be reasonable, for the purposes of informed decision making, to map these against crude estimates for prognosis, invasiveness of support, length of stay, the physical and mental burdens of weaning from support, the impact on subsequent overall health status, and future dependency on healthcare and medical interventions.

The most fundamental barrier to such decision making lies in the lack of prognostic accuracy, because there are very few conditions, such as brainstem death, that unequivocally allow practitioners to adopt an absolute position on outcome. Even if accurate survival figures were available, it is questionable, furthermore, whether an individual could or would make a choice to either accept or decline intensive care between a range of predicted mortality from very high to very low, because survival is an all-or-none phenomenon rather than relative. Systems have been devised to improve predictive accuracy and facilitate informed choice[15] and one would naturally incorporate factors such as age, comorbidity, and the reversibility of the triggering pathology into the prognosis and decision making, particularly if an individual scored highly across multiple fields, but it can be seen that these aspects, which inevitably lack precision for the individual patient, can rarely be determinative.

It could be considered reasonable, therefore, to eliminate these factors from the decision making and to base prognosis on the patient's response to escalation of care, recognizing the inherent difficulty of incorporating a deferred decision into the process of consent, which is founded on more precise and binding decision making while capacitous.

Are there issues beyond survival that are integral to consent, and can these be determined?

Not only is the prognosis for survival elusive for the individual patient for a particular set of circumstances, such that an actual trial of intensive care would be required for greater accuracy, but it is apparent that prognosis alone should not direct decision making. The likelihood of survival requires triangulation with the burden and length of intensive care, and the quality of life in the event of survival.

The concept of 'burden' is, however, both very individual and complex, because it covers not only pain and discomfort but also loss of autonomy and privacy, embarrassment at dependence on others for personal hygiene, innate objection to aspects of care such as catheterization, and fear of mental disturbance, any of which may skew a proactive decision when an individual is enjoying full health. It would be essential, therefore, to emphasize that many of these aspects are temporary and modifiable by medication to relieve discomfort, anxiety, or distress, and may actually be welcomed during critical illness as relief from the primary impact of that condition, a consideration that may not be apparent until that point in time. The experienced practitioner will thus have observed the patient with irreversible end-stage lung disease for whom all parties have consensually agreed on limiting support to non-invasive ventilation, but who then requests that intubation be reconsidered in the face of profound dyspnoea. It can be questioned, therefore, how any individual could prospectively and proactively assess the burdens of intensive care, or the burdens of rejecting invasive support, and generate a binding directive on this basis.

Quality of life in the event of survival is another highly subjective dimension, incorporating medically assessed markers such as organ dysfunction, neurological disability, and any predictable need for hospitalization or ongoing medical intervention but—more critically—considering the impact of these on the individual patient, their family, and relevant others. The patient would need to consider, therefore, aspects such as dependence on others, limitations in capacity for exercise or physical activity, restrictions on employment, social and leisure activity, the future viability of relationships, or any aspect that was of specific relevance and importance for that individual, and attempt to give these factors a more objective weighting when reaching an informed decision.

It is quite apparent that the overwhelming majority of individuals accommodate and adapt to significant illness and accompanying disability without considering an absence of value to their life, and it can be questioned, therefore, whether patients should be forced to make a decision proactively that may be skewed by their own and indeed their doctor's misconceptions as to the impact of disability, and consequently restrict their future access to life-sustaining medical treatment. It is acknowledged that there is very little data on longer-term outcomes from intensive care, with conflicting conclusions, certain studies suggesting greater levels of satisfaction among survivors than may have been predicted,[16] but with others questioning health-related quality of life.[17] It is also apparent that focused medical and psychological support programmes following discharge have the capacity to positively modify aspects of any recovery,[18] but provision of such care remains under-resourced and relatively random. In the face of inconsistent results and variability in access to appropriate treatment, it is difficult to imply to individual patients that this information should direct their decision.

A fundamental barrier to proactive consent is created, therefore, by the observation that the elements essential to an informed choice—prognosis, the burdens of intensive care, and quality of life in the event of survival—can only be determined more objectively by initiation of intensive care, a process that then prevents an informed choice by removing or significantly compromising an individual's capacity, and on this basis, making a truly informed choice again appear rarely possible.

Barriers to balanced communication on aspects of care

With lack of precision on key decision-making factors, one could argue that clinicians attempting proactive decision making should simply present information to the patient on the process of care, and simplify choice to refusal of intensive care or admission to intensive care with continuation of active treatment until absolute identification of medical futility. Although specific cases demonstrate how patients may have very consistent and fixed views on quality of life both prior and subsequent to intensive care, without the need for any such information on prognosis and treatment options, and prefer withdrawal of active support and death to the continuation of life-sustaining medical treatment (LSMT),[19] most practitioners would predictably feel uncomfortable offering such stark choices, and this strategy, while theoretically facilitating patient choice in certain cases, would not generally serve patient, professional, unit, or the broader public well.

In the face of uncertainty, a 'trial' of intensive care appears a pragmatic solution, but if subsequent decision making on the grounds of prognosis, the burdens of care, and quality of life in the event of survival cannot be based on pre-treatment discussion because the patient cannot take an informed view, and is therefore subsequently left to healthcare professionals and others once the process has been initiated, the process of consent is once again invalidated.

It is very difficult, furthermore, to present such complex information in a manner that can be understood both intellectually and emotionally, and is free from influence.

Most lay individuals would have difficulty understanding and processing detail on the complex components of care and the principles behind normalization of physiological systems, which theoretically is the most emotionally neutral aspect of the information. Even the description of these aspects has, however, the capacity to induce fear over the invasiveness, dependency, and loss of autonomy, which may then compromise rational decision making.

The communication of prognosis represents an even greater challenge, because simple issues such as whether this is described negatively, as in the risk of dying rather than the probability of survival, are likely to influence the response. It is known, for example, that mothers presented with a 20% risk of a Down's child are more likely to opt for amniocentesis than the group informed of an 80% chance of a normal child.[20] When the subject matter extends to debate on the burdens of intensive care and the quality of life in the event of survival, it is apparent that the topics are becoming more subjective and any overt emphasis on the negative aspects of care may be construed by the patient as an attempt to discourage uptake.

In these circumstances, there is the risk of the patient pursuing active care despite significant side effects and very little chance of survival, in the belief that the position of the healthcare professionals is driven by resource limitations or discrimination against certain categories of patient, rather than genuinely warning the patient and promoting an informed choice. One illustration of this is the higher likelihood of black American women opting for highly toxic chemotherapy with little chance of ensuring survival, based on the belief that the provision of information on this specific issue is designed to discourage them, being founded in persistent discrimination.[21]

While one would not expect such prejudice on the grounds of race or colour within contemporary intensive care, it is apparent that misconceptions or strongly held beliefs with regards to outcome from critical illness are present within the medical profession. Historically, there was a commonly held view that survival from an AIDS-defining illness requiring intensive care was so poor that admission was not indicated, until such time that outcome studies revealed otherwise.[22] Most practitioners will also acknowledge that nihilism over haematological malignancy, or a repeat admission for exacerbation of chronic obstructive pulmonary disease (COPD), will historically have skewed decision-making away from active support for these categories of patient.

The additional consideration that generates an uncomfortable element of decision making and is relevant to how information is given is the fact that intensive care is ultimately a limited geographical resource, and practitioners are routinely forced to consider which patients have the greatest chance of benefiting. While this should be based on clinical criteria without any discrimination or consideration of an individual's worth to society, there are occasions, such as an admission veto of the decompensated Jehovah's Witness who is refusing all blood products, that might be construed by others as discrimination on religious grounds.

It is important to acknowledge, therefore, that factors other than the patient's best interests may influence communication with the patient or their next of kin, such as resource limitations or the practitioner's preconceptions, and even in the absence of these issues the dialogue may unduly influence a decision, either because emphasis is placed on negative aspects or religious and cultural views are not recognized or accommodated, generating a request for all active support despite clear evidence of futility, based on a belief that discrimination is driving decision making.

There are significant barriers, therefore, to providing understandable information on the process and complexity of intensive care, which raise additional questions as to whether proactive consent can ever be achieved. A further problem is generated because, theoretically, a patient should not be forced to refuse or sign up to the package of care that is the standard for the individual unit, but should be able to access a style of care that approximates to their own values and beliefs. If, however, the process of care becomes fragmented with certain aspects of care declined, delivery of the overall goals may be significantly compromised, in addition to the obvious practical problems in providing piecemeal care. If, furthermore, intensive care is reduced to a definable package, dictated by consent, there would inevitably be restrictions on refining techniques and introducing new technology, or trialling new treatment options in the face of a poor response to first-line treatment. The question has to be asked, therefore, whether the patient can and should be allowed any autonomy regarding particular facets of intensive care.

Aspects of care that benefit others

Certain aspects of care are not directed specifically at individual patient benefit but reflect either an obligation to utilize the resource effectively and efficiently, or broader professional goals such as audit and research. It is questionable whether these factors, which either bring no individual benefit or actually compromise patient well-being can be considered an integral component of the package that in effect the patient consents to when agreeing to intensive care. For example, if the policy of an intensive care unit (ICU) is to transfer the most stable and least dependent patient out when demand exceeds availability, is the prospective patient in any position to refuse this option proactively, and can a lack of objection at the outset be viewed as adequate consent when the need arises for such transfer? Similarly, if research or the education of medical students is the norm for a specific unit, is it possible for a patient to prospectively opt out without harbouring concerns that commitment to their care will be compromised, and therefore feel under obligation to consent?

Other related issues include organ donation and post-mortem examinations that cause a high level of angst among next of kin in the usual circumstances of facing difficult decisions without any true inkling of the patient's position on these matters.

While clearly it would assist both practitioners and next of kin in subsequent discussions if the patient's opinion was known, there are potential harms of induced anxiety if the patient, in an already vulnerable state, considers either that a 'positive' response to donation may skew the process of care away from making every effort to preserve life and more towards the potential recipient, or regarding a post-mortem, that death is the likely outcome.

Capacity—elusive and potentially harmful

A further problem in the pursuit of consent is created by the varying and unpredictable levels of capacity at various stages of a critical illness, because consent is intended to be a dynamic process with the opportunity for revision at any stage, and theoretically moments of competence should be used to confirm or cancel the patient's previously expressed position, or establish their position if a previous determination has not been reached.

The reality is that capacity is invariably compromised in these circumstances, creating the burden of the decision-making process for the patient while simultaneously questioning the validity of that decision making and undermining the value of the exercise. Although the Mental Capacity Act 2005 specifies the continuous assessment of capacity and the need to promote capacity whenever this is compromised, the usual scenario within intensive care is that a genuinely capacitous state is rarely reached, and harms can be created by efforts to ensure this if analgesia and sedation are withdrawn solely to assess capacity, by generating discomfort and distress, which themselves compromise capacity. If, therefore, there are significant barriers to achieving informed consent prior to or within the early stages of a critical illness before capacity is compromised, and this becomes even less attainable once the critical illness is established, how can the principle of respect for autonomy be practically applied?

Patients' views and wishes

This raises the more fundamental question of whether consent as a process for life-sustaining medical treatment [LSMT] is something that patients really wish to engage in proactively. In those jurisdictions where advance directives have a formal status, only a small percentage of the population have completed such an order, believing this to be restrictive on future choices by failing to anticipate either advances in medical care or indeed changes of the patient's perceptions once acute illness supervened. In these circumstances, patients expressed a preference for 'benign medical paternalism', which accommodated the ongoing opinion of the next of kin as representative of the patient's values and beliefs.[23] It is important, therefore, to distinguish acceptable variants of benign medical paternalism from the discredited examples of withholding information to protect patients and relatives from distressing details. This approach generated significant public distrust in the medical profession in the aftermath of the Alder Hey retained organs scandal and was instrumental in change to the determination of a patient's resuscitation status, with the current expectation that the patient be given the ultimate authority.

This does of course raise the issue of whether the patient is better served by being invited as a consumer to make a choice on a complex subject of which predictably they would have limited knowledge, and in the circumstances of hospitalization and illness that carry the hazard of compromising rational decision making, with potential automatic exclusion of medical advice. The benign medical paternalism that is seemingly sought by patients incorporates the therapeutic value of taking decisions when requested to, and assisting decision making with advice and recommendations when similarly requested, without compromising an individual's need for control in certain key areas. This construct accommodates a full spectrum of patients' wishes, from the individual who wishes to make their own informed choice to those who wish not to be given information on treatment options and who prefer medical guidance. While appearing at first visit to be contrary to contemporary ethical principles, this construct clearly seeks to determine the patient's wishes with regards to levels of patient–practitioner responsibility for decision making, and retains the service facet of the doctor–patient relationship, with value and reassurance for patient as well as practitioner and public. It would be regrettable if the majority of the population were disadvantaged by imperatives driven by worthy principles but enforced by a small minority who simplistically demand that the position of the patient is determinative.

The status of the next of kin in decision making

A further confounding factor in whatever approach is taken towards consent is the status of the next of kin in decision making once the patient loses capacity. While most members of the public would be confident that their values and beliefs would be accurately represented by their next of kin, their authority is limited to providing information on these aspects, unless formally empowered with a lasting power of attorney for personal welfare (LPAPW) with specified responsibility regarding LSMT. Although government directives and professional guidelines specify the involvement of the next of kin in decision making for the incompetent patient, their ability to direct care will therefore be limited. The ideal scenario for patient care in these circumstances is an absolute consensus position from intensive care team, parent specialty and next of kin, and in the majority of cases this is achieved without placing any responsibility for decision making on the next of kin, a position that should be avoided. Transferring responsibility onto the next of kin for a decision in an area where their expertise is limited and where their emotional involvement could inappropriately compromise objectivity, carries the risk of longer-term guilt or resentment towards healthcare staff if they believe themselves responsible for either limiting LSMT prematurely or, alternatively, forcing the burden of protracted ineffective support on the patient. The converse of this is when the opinion of the next of kin as to the appropriate course of action is ignored, and, if patients have no faith in medical decision making or the concept of benign medical paternalism, there is little alternative to a highly specific advance directive or appointment of a LPAPW in ensuring that one's wishes are both explicit and determinative.

Pragmatic solutions

In the face of the above problems, it would be understandable if intensive care staff considered proactive consent too elusive a concept and reverted to a historical model whereby patients were admitted under the parent specialty as a continuum of acute care, with little anticipatory engagement by the intensive care team. The reality is, however, that intensive care carries a high mortality rate and, with the exception of those patients who demonstrate a spiral of deterioration refractory to all treatment strategies, decisions will have to be taken on the continuation of active support when it becomes apparent for whatever reason that the goals of intensive care are not attainable.

In these circumstances, all relevant parties are protected if the decision making is as informed as possible by the patient's values and beliefs with regard to dependency on medical support, tolerable quality of life in the event of survival, and position on what constitutes a good death. It appears inescapable therefore that, when circumstances suggest a high likelihood of requiring intensive care, these issues should be explored and formally documented. It should also be apparent that, even when survival is the more likely outcome, intensive care is invasive and associated with significant physical and psychological burdens, potentially over a protracted period. For this to be justifiable, there has to be strong evidence that this approximates to the patient's wishes. It is also clear that failing to proactively engage the patient causes broader individual and societal harms. If the patient is not made aware of the seriousness of their condition before the point of decompensation, they are denied the opportunity to plan for dying and, if patients are denied the opportunity to decline admission to intensive care, then not only is this cohort of patients inappropriately managed with little respect for autonomy but a hardship is also imposed on the public by unwarranted expense and a restriction on access to a scarce resource for those patients more capable of benefiting.

This exercise has to be undertaken therefore and, although much of the primary information and opinion gathering can be undertaken by the parent specialty, it requires a member of the intensive care team to facilitate an informed discussion on the benefits and risks of intensive care. This approach is in line with the principles of consent for other medical and surgical activity, where it is anticipated that the practitioner undertaking the consent process is someone capable of delivering the proposed care or intervention. The opportunity for early engagement of patient and family outside the geographical confines of the ICU already exists, via the platform of outreach critical care, at the point when Early Warning Scores trigger assessments at ward level. This evaluation can reasonably progress beyond recommending strategies to rectifying physiological derangement and asking, 'Does this patient require an ICU admission?', 'Will this patient benefit from an ICU admission?' and 'Does this patient want an ICU admission?'. Such an assessment requires a determination on capacity in the first instance, followed by an appraisal of the impact of comorbidity and medical interventions on background quality of life, focusing when appropriate on when these factors would make life intolerable and when therefore the patient would not wish to undergo LSMT. Even if a decision is taken to escalate care, it is important to have this information as an objective point of reference should complications develop that would take the patient across the specified threshold and into the 'intolerable burden of living' territory. This condition demands that a patient's higher neurological function is grossly intact such that they are aware of their condition and thereby suffer, a situation that most intensive care patients are protected from. Ultimately, this assessment has then to be undertaken by others, thereby once more compromising principles of consent or placing an undue burden on the next of kin to provide a 'substituted judgement', but this is at least assisted by an earlier exploration with the patient.

An additional concern of the public is profound neurological disability, which, even if not associated with suffering, represents loss of identity and dignity, and constitutes a burden to others, such that many individuals would not wish to be maintained with LSMT if there was no chance of a meaningful recovery from their perspective. These aspects should certainly be discussed if proposed interventions such as intra-cranial surgery or major vascular procedures carry a risk of neurological insult.

Having explored the above areas, it would then be reasonable to determine how active a participant in healthcare decision making the patient wished to be. Respect for autonomy does not translate into simply providing information and expecting the patient to decide, but offering a range of options including making a choice with limited information or asking the doctor to make recommendations based on knowledge of the disease, potential treatments, and the health status and values of the patient. Respect for autonomy may also include accommodating the patient's wishes that no decisions be made at that point in time, but, in the event of requiring intensive care at some future point and not fulfilling the criteria for capacity, that decisions be taken between medical staff and next of kin.

Meeting the expectations of patients, given this range of attitudes and wishes, is clearly problematical, and requires detailed information on the process of care, outcomes, the staff involved, decision making for the incompetent adult, the role of the next of kin, sharing of information, research, etc. for those patients who wish to make as informed a decision as possible. It can be anticipated that most patients would only wish for overview information on these issues rather than highly specific detail, and it is possible, therefore, to have basic information booklets with the option of secondary pamphlets on aspects that would be of particular interest to the patient, such as transfusion or a tracheostomy.

It is also important to distinguish between the main categories of patient who would predictably approach these difficult questions differently. Those patients who carry a high risk of decompensation in association with elective surgery should theoretically be better placed to address these questions rationally without the adverse influence of ill health, and a determination of their wishes on key issues can reasonably be pursued. It has to be considered, however, that extensive discussion on the limitations and harms of intensive care may not be ideal mental preparation for major surgery from the patient's perspective.

Patients whose background pathology will predictably require intensive care at some future stage if life is to be sustained, such as advanced respiratory disease or neurodegenerative disorders, should also be engaged as soon as feasible, given the predictably worse outcome within this cohort of patients compared with 'elective' admissions. These undertakings should be the responsibility of the parent specialty as specified by the regulatory body in relation to patients with progressive disease and a life expectancy of 12 months or fewer,[24] but most intensive care practitioners would predictably declare that they find very little evidence of this obligation being fulfilled.

Patients who are admitted acutely and on the verge of decompensation at the point an ICU assessment is requested are likely to be less capable of and willing to undergo a demanding series of questions on quality of life and values and beliefs, and staff should therefore be mindful of pursuing otherwise ideal goals. In these circumstances, engagement of the next of kin is essential, acknowledging that at a time of significant distress it will predictably be difficult to consolidate information on illness, prognosis, process of care, and the limitations on their authority for decision making.

It can also be anticipated that next of kin will not always be in agreement with the medical overview and recommendations, particularly if these favour a limitation on active support. This may be due to understandable factors such as an unwillingness to take responsibility for such a significant decision within a relatively pressurized time frame, or a genuinely held belief that the patient's quality of life was acceptable despite major disability. Other drivers for a contrary position include guilt over their previous commitment to care and support of the patient, religious views on the sanctity of life, or a belief that the medical position is driven by discrimination on the grounds of age, lifestyle, or religion, or that resource allocation is a primary concern. In these circumstances, although the emphasis has to be on protecting the patient from the harms of interventions that will be futile from either a physiological perspective or because they will not restore an acceptable quality of life, the patient's best interests are rarely promoted by conflict between healthcare team and next of kin. Maintaining communication, exploring the drivers behind an individual's position, empathizing with their circumstances, allowing time and space, and making concessions are important strategies in maintaining both dialogue and mutual respect, which in turn are fundamental to concepts of consent. Although recognizing that in extreme circumstances an application to the courts might be essential to resolve an impasse that is generating obvious patient harms, a process that pits the relative authority of healthcare professionals and the legal system against the next of kin who by definition are in a vulnerable position, intuitively runs contrary to broad principles of consent.

An aspect of intensive care responsibilities that is often overlooked in these discussions with either patient or next of kin relates to end-of-life procedures when ICU admission is not considered, or when a later decision is taken to withdraw active support when the goals of intensive care have not been realized. The public are only too aware of how even UK doctors feel that they have to end their lives overseas in pursuit of a good death,[25] and would predictably wish for reassurance that any discomfort or distress associated with dying would be managed competently and confidently without fear of professional repercussions. It is apparent that there is a range of practice in this area[26] and a restrictive approach borne out of the practitioner's personal beliefs should engender greater public concern than benign paternalism. Unit policy and practice on these issues should therefore be unambiguous and accessible, with the overall benefit of protecting all parties. This responsibility to promote and provide a 'good death' when this is inevitable extends equally to those patients who are refused or who decline ICU admission, because this is an integral part of the overall responsibility and decision-making process, particularly when palliative care may not be able to accommodate the patient within a reasonable time frame.

There may therefore be many facets to consent and many barriers to approaching an ideal model, but policies need to be formulated to meet the needs of particular institutions and to demonstrate that the principles of legislation such as the Mental Capacity Act are being adhered to. The process of patient engagement on these issues needs documentation to confirm compliance with all directives, but more importantly as an objective point of reference on the patient's quality of life, values, and beliefs, which will shape medical decision making once the patient has lost capacity and the goals of intensive care are not achievable.

National initiatives covering exploration, discussion, and documentation on values and beliefs are underway in the form of the ReSPECT process (Recommended Summary Plan For Emergency Care And Treatment),[1] with the increasing adoption by healthcare organizations. Whilst this represents a conceptual and practical refinement of the previous determination of resuscitation status, and incorporates certain of the principles of proactive/pre-emptive engagement, it remains the opinion of this author that the initiative does not and cannot address many of the problematical areas highlighted above.

Conclusions

Consent, the cornerstone of contemporary medical practice, is a challenging concept when considering the complexities of intensive care. To achieve the maximum good for all parties, this political and professional imperative has to go beyond simple provision of information, patient choice, and documentation of process. The majority of patients requiring intensive care may be better served by broad discussion of their values and goals, an ongoing evaluation of their response to escalating interventions and cares, and delayed decision making informed by these aspects, predictably when the patient has lost capacity. Whilst this approach may be criticized as paternalism, however benign, it appears preferable to early forced patient choice, which superficially would conform with political directives but which carries the risk of simplistic decisions that then restrict future choice. If we are to offer options as an essential feature of consent, these should arguably include that of allowing the healthcare team to take decisions once the patient loses capacity, in the light of their response to treatment.

These approaches may be viewed, however, as contravening current standards of consent by individuals or organizations unfamiliar with the complexities of intensive care, and the whole subject needs broad professional and public debate therefore if we are to achieve maximal patient and public good, limit practitioner vulnerabilities, and enhance the status of

---

[1] https://www.resus.org.uk/respect/

our specialty by demonstrating a reasoned and reasonable strategy in this challenging area.

References

1. *Montgomery v Lanarkshire Health Board* [2015] SC 11 [2015] 1 AC 1430.
2. https://www.england.nhs.uk/nhs-standard-contract/cquin (accessed 25 November 2019).
3. *The Report of the Inquiry into children's heart surgery at the Bristol Royal Infirmary 1984–1995: Learning from Bristol.* (2001). (Cm 5207). The Stationery Office, London.
4. Redfern M. (2001). *The Royal Liverpool Children's Inquiry Report.* The Stationery Office, London.
5. http://www.legislation.gov.uk/ukpga/2004/30/contents (accessed 25 November 2019).
6. *Chester v Afshar* [2004] HL 41. http://www.publications.parliament.uk/pa/ld200304/ldjudgmt/jd041014/cheste-1.htm (accessed 25 November 2019).
7. Department of Health (2009). *Reference guide to consent for examination or treatment*, 4th edn. Department of Health https://assets.publishing.service.gov.uk/government/uploads/system/uploads/attachment_data/file/138296/dh_103653_ _1_.pdf (accessed 25 November 2019).
8. General Medical Council (2008). *Consent: patients and doctors making decisions together.* General Medical Council.
9. http://www.opsi.gov.uk/acts/acts2005/ukpga_20050009_en_1 (accessed 25 November 2019).
10. NHS Executive (2000). *HSC 2000/028. Resuscitation Policy.* Department of Health, London.
11. https://www.sccm.org/SurvivingSepsisCampaign/Home (accessed 30 December 2019).
12. https://www.cochrane.org/CD002042/INJ_it-safe-use-lower-blood-counts-trigger-blood-transfusion-order-give-fewer-blood-transfusions (accessed 25 November 2019).
13. Andriolo BN, et al. (2015). *Early versus late tracheostomy for critically ill patients.* Cochrane Database Systemic Review.
14. Subbe CP, Kruger M, Rutherford P, Gemmel L. (2001). Validation of a Modified Early Warning Score in medical admissions. *Q J Med*, **94**, 521–6.
15. Knaus WA, Harrell FE Jr, Lynn J, et al. (1995). The SUPPORT prognostic model. Objective estimates of survival for seriously ill hospitalized adults. Study to

understand prognoses and preferences for outcomes and risks of treatments. *Ann Intern Med*, 1 Feb, **122**(3), 191–203.

16. Eddleston JM, White P, Guthrie E. (2000). Survival, morbidity, and quality-of-life after discharge from intensive care. *Critical Care Medicine*, **28**(7), 2293–9.

17. Hofhuis JG, Spronk PE, van Stel HF, et al. (2008). The impact of critical illness on perceived health related quality-of-life during ICU treatment, hospital stay, and after hospital discharge; a long term follow-up study. *Chest*, **133**, 377–85.

18. Cuthbertson BH, Rattray J, Johnston M, et al. (2007). A pragmatic randomised, controlled trial of intensive care follow up programmes in improving longer-term outcomes from critical illness: the PRACTICAL study. *BMC Health Serv Res*, 7, 116.

19. *Ms B v An NHS Hospital Trust* [2002] EWHC 429 (Fam).

20. McNeil BJ, Pauker SG, Sox HC, Tversky A. (1982). On elicitation of preferences for alternative therapies. *N Engl J Med*, **306**, 1259–62.

21. Lerner BH. (2001). *The breast cancer wars. Hope, fear and the pursuit of a cure in twentieth-century America*. Oxford University Press, New York.

22. Bhagwanjee S, et al. (1997). Does HIV status influence the outcome of patients admitted to a surgical intensive care unit? A prospective double blind study. *BMJ*, **314**, 1077–84.

23. Perkins HS. (2007). Controlling death: the false promise of advance directives. *Ann Intern Med*, **147**, 51–7.

24. General Medical Council. (2010). *Treatment and care towards the end of life: good practice in decision making*. General Medical Council, London.

25. Obituaries. Anne Turner. (2010). *British Medical Journal*, **332**, 306.

26. Poulton B, Ridley S, Mackenzie-Ross R, Rizvi S. (2005). Variation in end-of-life decision-making between critical care consultants. *Anaesthesia*, **60**, 1101–5.

2

Refusing and Demanding Medical Treatment in Intensive Care

Alex Ruck Keene and Zoë Fritz

Introduction: setting the scene

The intensive care unit (ICU) is the scene of clinicians summoning machines and medications to support multiple organs that are failing. These so-called 'heroic measures' can increase the prospects of survival for critically ill patients[1] but those who survive can be left with impaired physical or mental function, or with psychological damage.[2] Clinicians are driven by the desire to save lives, but must also ensure that they uphold the Hippocratic tenant of '*Primum non nocere*'.[3] In the context of a patient demanding or refusing a treatment on the ICU, clinicians need to understand what might constitute harm for that individual patient; have appropriately communicated the risks of having (or not having) the treatment; understand the professional guidance and ethical framework in which decisions are made, and know the law and how it might constrain (or allow) them to act in certain ways.

Having set the scene, this chapter then looks in detail at the interactions between adult patients with capacity and the clinical team as regards the refusal of, or requests for, specific treatments. It also addresses the position of such a patient seeking to project forward their decisions by way of advance decisions to refuse treatment. The positions of the adult patient without capacity and that of children are dealt with in Chapters 5 and 4 respectively, although we touch on the former here in a number of places to draw contrasts with the position of the (apparently) autonomous adult patient with capacity.

Constituting harm and communicating risk

Although we have used the term 'refusing and demanding treatment' in the chapter heading, we note immediately that the term is in itself incendiary: it pits patient against clinician, infantilizing the patient and projecting a stern, authoritarian stance on the clinician. In fact the law, professional guidance, and ethical norms all suggest that clinicians and patients (or those close to them) should work together to determine what treatments might be beneficial to the patient. This is not an easy step for several reasons.

1. It is hard to convey the reality of what treatments on the ICU entail to those who have never been inside one. Researchers have compiled patients' and relatives' stories on Healthtalk[4] and a charity called 'ICUsteps' has compiled a patient information leaflet in liaison with the Department of Health (now the Department of Health and Social Care).[5] A video conveying what happens in attempted cardiopulmonary resuscitation (CPR) led to greater patient understanding than pictures and words alone,[6] and perhaps such videos should be made for explaining what treatments occur on an ICU. As an indicator of what truly 'informed' patients might want, it is interesting to note that many American physicians would not want the level of intensive treatments that they give to their patients because they feel many of them are harmful.[7]

2. It is hard for clinicians to translate population risks into individual risk and also hard to communicate the uncertainty in outcome.[8] When offering or withholding a treatment, a doctor is legally bound to communicate the 'material risks' of the treatment offered, and any reasonable alternatives. This was emphasized by the Supreme Court in *Montgomery v Lanarkshire Health Board*:

   The doctor is [...] under a duty to take reasonable care to ensure that the patient is aware of any material risks involved in any recommended treatment, and of any reasonable alternative or variant treatments. The test of materiality is whether, in the circumstances of the particular case, a reasonable person in the patient's position would be likely to attach significance to the risk, or the doctor is or should reasonably be aware that the particular patient would be likely to attach significance to it.[9]

   In the context of an acutely sick patient who needs urgent, often emergency, treatment decisions, the time available to discuss the risks of different treatment options in a comprehensible way is severely limited.

3. It is hard for patients to balance a risk of survival in a severely diminished state with the risk of survival with good function and the risk of

death, and having a conversation about this at a time of acute illness makes it even harder.

One proposed solution for this that has been under development since 2014 has been to concentrate not on which *treatments* might be desired or feared, but instead to focus on what *outcomes* the patient values. The ReSPECT process[10] helps patients and doctors have conversations in advance of an acute illness, guiding them through understanding patients' preferences and then recording clinical recommendations that can be easily recognized in an emergency. While patients may, of course, change their minds when faced with the actual possibility of death without treatment, having this conversation in advance can prepare them for revisiting it, and provides clinicians with a starting point in the event of the patient lacking capacity. However, when the patient is requesting a treatment that the doctor believes will cause them harm, or refusing one that the doctor believes they will benefit from, the doctor must draw on professional guidance, ethical analysis, and the law to know how to respond.

How do professional guidance, ethical analysis, and the law interact?

Professional guidance, ethical argument, and the law sometimes pull in different directions, and sometimes inform each other.[11] Professional guidance—such as that published by the General Medical Council (GMC)[12]—lays out the 'professional values and behaviours expected from any doctor registered'. Such guidance is updated regularly in response to new challenges doctors face both clinically and interpersonally. It incorporates current case law and legislation, but sometimes this guidance goes further: such guidance is often referred to in court as a reflection of current best practice. Empirical ethics research and ethical analysis can reveal flaws in current practice and force clinicians and patients to challenge current norms. The law exists to protect liberties and rights, but, in doing so, can unintentionally change behaviour in other ways.[13] In *Winspear v City Hospitals Sunderland NHS FT*,[14] for example, it was held that, in a situation where a patient lacked capacity and an advance resuscitation decision had to be made, clinicians should contact those close to the patient as long as it was 'practicable and appropriate' to do so. Despite the (intentional) nuance in the language of this judgment, discussed further in Chapter 3, clinicians are now driven by what may well be a misplaced fear

of litigation into doing what sometimes feels ethically wrong: phoning up elderly people, who live too far away to come to the hospital, in the middle of the
night to ask if they have any knowledge of their relative's wishes regarding
resuscitation.

While the law on discussing resuscitation decisions is now clear, the ex-
trapolation of this law into decisions about referring or admitting to the ICU
has not yet been tested in court. Further, and perhaps because of the difficulty
in explaining the range of treatments and risks, decisions about treatments
on the ICU are still often made without full consultation with the patient
and (where the patient lacks capacity) those close to them,[15] or 'choices'
are presented in such a way that does not so much nudge the patient down
a particular path but leaves them no other viable option. In these situations,
clinicians most frequently sees themselves as using their 'clinical judgment
and experience' to make the 'right decision', often balancing competing demands on resources for other patients as well.

It is in situations like this and others where, either because the process of
discussion has been curtailed as inadequate or because of some other factor,
the patient does not see eye to eye with the doctors, that terms such as 'demanding and refusing treatment' emerge and the law in this area is called into
action: even if, as we discuss in the next section, the law is built on important,
but possibly questionable, fictions about patients.

Refusal of treatment

Contemporaneous refusal of treatment

The law in England and Wales has created the concept of the autonomous patient, with sovereignty over their own body. That sovereignty is not complete,
obvious exceptions being in relation to children, those subject to the Mental
Health Act 1983, and those held to lack decision-making capacity. As we will
see, the law has also carved out a legally clear but (in practice) sometimes
practically difficult exception in relation to those subject to undue influence
or coercion. As we will also see, the concept of the autonomous patient starts
to crumble significantly when looked at closely.

Decisions both pre- and post-dating the Mental Capacity Act 2005 ('MCA
2005') have made clear how strongly the courts are willing to defend the
concept of the autonomous patient in the context of the delivery of potentially life-saving treatment.[16] By way of example, in *Re B*,[17] the court was
concerned with a professional woman in her forties, who became paralyzed

from the neck down as a result of a cervical cavernoma. She could move her head and use some of her neck muscles but she could not move her torso, arms, and legs at all. She was totally dependent on her carers in the ICU where she had been for a year. Her life was supported by artificial ventilation. Without it, she would have a less than 1% chance of independent ventilation, and death would almost certainly follow. She wanted the ventilator turned off but her doctors refused to do so. She brought proceedings in the Family Division of the High Court seeking declarations that she had the mental capacity to choose whether or not to accept the treatment and that the hospital was treating her unlawfully, together with nominal damages to recognize the tort of trespass to her person. Granting her the remedies that she sought, Dame Elizabeth Butler-Sloss P, the then-President of the Family Division, held that:

> If mental capacity is not in issue and the patient, having been given the relevant information and offered the available options, chooses to refuse the treatment, that decision has to be respected by the doctors. Considerations that the best interests of the patient would indicate that the decision should be to consent to treatment are irrelevant.

And, further, that:

> The treating clinicians and the hospital should always have in mind that a seriously physically disabled patient who is mentally competent has the same right to personal autonomy and to make decisions as any other person with mental capacity.[18]

More recently, MacDonald J in *Kings College Hospital NHS Foundation Trust v C*[19] (a case concerning refusal of life-sustaining renal haemodialysis by a woman following an attempt to take her own life) held that:

> The court being satisfied that, in accordance with the provisions of the Mental Capacity Act 2005, C has capacity to decide whether or not to accept treatment C is entitled to make her own decision on that question based on the things that are important to her, in keeping with her own personality and system of values and without conforming to society's expectation of what constitutes the 'normal' decision in this situation (if such a thing exists). As a capacitous individual C is, in respect of her own body and mind, sovereign.

As these cases make clear, the courts emphasize the extent to which capacity is a gateway (in this context) to the exercise of autonomy. However, both at the level of high legal principle and in practice, *how* capacity in this context actually applies is not always straightforward.

Before the MCA 2005 was enacted, the courts had proceeded on the basis that there was a sliding scale of capacity to refuse medical treatment—the 'more serious the decision, the greater the capacity required'.[20] However, there is no such scale in the MCA itself, the question always falling to be determined on the balance of probabilities.[21] MacDonald J in the *C* case also emphasized that 'the *outcome* of the decision made is not relevant to the question of whether the person taking the decision has capacity for the purposes of the Mental Capacity Act 2005' (emphasis added).[22]

The courts have also routinely spoken of the need to secure against the 'protection' imperative, emphasizing that:

> the temptation to base a judgment of a person's capacity upon whether they seem to have made a good or bad decision, and in particular on whether they have accepted or rejected medical advice, is absolutely to be avoided. That would be to put the cart before the horse or, expressed another way, to allow the tail of welfare to wag the dog of capacity. Any tendency in this direction risks infringing the rights of that group of persons who, though vulnerable, are capable of making their own decisions. Many who suffer from mental illness are well able to make decisions about their medical treatment, and it is important not to make unjustified assumptions to the contrary.[23]

These statements represent a particular—legal—conception of autonomy that is deeply engrained in the lawyers and judges applying the MCA 2005: the right of an individual, acting in isolation, to say 'no'. This version of autonomy enshrined in the cases set out earlier reflects (but is not directly drawn from) a similar version that holds very considerable weight among medical ethicists.[24] However, other scholars, from different disciplines, have increasingly questioned (1) whether it is not predicated upon a very 'thin' conception of autonomy that does not properly take into account the extent to which individuals do not make decisions in isolation,[25] and (2) the extent to which the absence of other choices may ultimately compel people to refuse treatments out of sense of desperation.[26]

Indeed, in one view, the extracts from the judgments set out earlier might be seen just as much exhortatory as anything else. Judges, no less than clinicians, find it remarkably difficult to escape the gravitational pull of the protection imperative when a person is refusing life-sustaining treatment for 'bad' reasons.[27] Indeed, although the courts have consistently sought to emphasize that a person, with capacity, can refuse for any reason, whether good, bad, or non-existent,[28] it is telling how often the judges seek to find a reason that they can understand. In *Ms B's* case, Dame Elizabeth Butler-Sloss was at pains to identify the strength of Ms B's will (and to seek, by her judgment, to persuade Ms B to change her mind); in similar vein, in the *C* case, MacDonald J rooted C's decision in the singularly (on the face of it, possibly pathologically) self-centred nature of her personality, as relayed by her daughters in their evidence to the court.

A very specific subset of such cases involves those who refuse treatment (or forms of treatment) on religious grounds, and it is striking how judges have sought to differentiate between situations in which a person with a mental health condition is refusing medical treatment on the basis of a 'conventional' religious belief and situations in which they are refusing such treatment on the basis of an idiosyncratic belief system. In the case of *Nottinghamshire Healthcare NHS Trust v RC*, for instance, Mostyn J was undoubtedly strongly influenced in his conclusion that a declaration should be granted that blood transfusions should not be administered under the compulsory provisions of the Mental Health Act 1983 to a detained patient seriously self-harming himself by the fact that the man in question sought to refuse such treatment—and to make an advance decision refusing such treatment—on the basis of his profession of faith as a Jehovah's Witness. As Mostyn J noted, 'It would be an extreme example of the application of the law of unintended consequences were an iron tenet of an accepted religion to give rise to questions of capacity under the MCA.'[29] By contrast, in *Wye Valley*, a factor contributing to Peter Jackson J's conclusion that the man in question (who had persistent and treatment-resistant schizoaffective disorder) lacked capacity to decide whether to have his leg amputated was that he heard angelic voices that told him whether or not to take his medication in the context of an unconventional belief system.[30] It is clear from the judgment that Peter Jackson J felt more comfortable accommodating the religious sentiments that were 'extremely important' to the man through the prism of best interests, and one of the factors that he took into account in deciding that the amputation should not proceed was that the man told him, 'I'm not afraid of dying, I know where I'm going. The angels have told me I am going to heaven. I have no regrets. It would be a better life than this.'[31]

Alongside, but at a complex tangent to the concept of capacity as the gateway to the exercise of autonomy, is the concept of vulnerability, which the courts use as they strain to find ways in which to ensure the protection of those patients who appear to be under the influence of third parties. Before the MCA 2005, the need to identify whether such a patient lacked capacity to refuse, or had capacity but was under duress, was not so important, because in either case the High Court could grant so-called declaratory relief.[32] Subsequent to the enactment of the MCA 2005, it has become *legally* important, if clinically complex, to identify whether the root cause of a person's apparently unwise refusal is down to the effects of an impairment or disturbance in their mind or brain or to the effects of the influence of a third party.[33] If the former, then the person will lack capacity, and treatment could be provided if such is in their best interests. If the latter, then the person does not lack capacity and, if a satisfactory agreement cannot be resolved on the ground in the unit, recourse to the somewhat ill-charted waters of the High Court's inherent jurisdiction will be needed.[34] Here, again, the interaction between the highly individualistic (dare one say 'atomistic') idea of mental capacity and the reality of decision making in the context of the individual's familial and social circumstances pose challenges that are as much ethical as they are strictly legal.[35]

Where in this mix does the concept of feeling like 'being a burden' sit? This is a familiar concept to many in the clinical setting, but one that the law finds difficult to address. In legal terms, unless the person is being (overly) influenced in their belief by the actions of a third party, or the belief is such as to render them incapable of making a decision within the meaning of the MCA 2005, then refusing treatment on the basis that the person considers that they are a burden, either to their family or more broadly to society, is a refusal that has to be accepted by the clinicians. In an intriguing passage in his judgment in the *Nicklinson* case[36] Lord Sumption (perhaps inadvertently) posed the question as to *why* such a refusal should be accepted. This case arose in a—legally—entirely different context, namely assisted dying, but in the context of giving reasons as to why he considered the Supreme Court should not involve itself in determining whether assisted dying should be made legal, Lord Sumption noted that:

> even the mentally competent may have reasons for deciding to kill themselves which reflect either overt pressure upon them by others or their own assumptions about what others may think or expect. The difficulty is particularly acute in the case of what the Commission on Assisted Dying called 'indirect social pressure'. This refers to the problems arising from the low self-esteem of many old or severely ill and dependent people, combined with the spontaneous and negative perceptions of patients about the views of those around them. The great majority of people contemplating suicide for health-related reasons, are likely to be acutely conscious that their disabilities make them dependent on others. These disabilities may arise from illness or injury, or indeed (a much larger category) from the advancing infirmity of old age. People in this position are vulnerable. They are often afraid that their lives have become a burden to those around them. The fear may be the result

of overt pressure, but may equally arise from a spontaneous tendency to place a low value on their own lives and assume that others do so too. Their feelings of uselessness are likely to be accentuated in those who were once highly active and engaged with those around them, for whom the contrast between now and then must be particularly painful. These assumptions may be mistaken but are none the less powerful for that. [...] *It is one thing to assess someone's mental ability to form a judgment, but another to discover their true reasons for the decision which they have made and to assess the quality of those reasons*[37] (emphasis added).

Of course, there may be individuals who have a strong sense of self-worth, but whose autonomous choice is that they would no longer wish to continue living if they reached a stage where they would consider themselves a burden. While it is impossible to disentangle the societal pressures and values systems in which these views develop, it is reasonable to argue that an individual's interests extend beyond their own personhood: a parent may wish a child to be able to live their life free of the duties of caring for a physically dependent and cognitively diminished relative.

There is no logical reason to consider that the pressures that Lord Sumption identifies are not equally at work when a person is refusing treatment, and the passage from his judgment undoubtedly poses a challenge to the model of autonomy described above. Indeed, if we take the example of one specific form of treatment refusal, namely ventilator removal in the context of those with motor neurone disease (MND), we can see that clinical guidance already seeks to guide clinicians to question the 'true reasons' for the decision that has been made. In detailed guidance drawn up by the Association for Palliative Medicine (APM) addressing ventilator removal at the request of those with MND,[38] a section on 'validating the decision' directs a senior doctor that they need to ensure that the request is 'a settled decision of a patient with capacity', and, in documenting the decision to proceed with withdrawal and evaluating the decision, suggests that the doctor should record, inter alia, that:

- the alternative approaches are known and rejected by the patient
- the patient knows they will die as a consequence of withdrawal
- there is no coercion, *nor is the decision driven by mistaken kindness to the family* (emphasis added)
- this [is] a settled view of the patient.

The guidance leaves tantalizingly open what should happen if the doctor takes the view that the decision *is* driven by mistaken kindness to the family. Lord Sumption would—perhaps—suggest that the decision should not be honoured, but the logic of the case law set out at the start of this section is to directly contrary effect.

Ventilation, and ventilation refusal, also points to a further area where apparently clear legal principles rub up awkwardly against clinical reality, and the reality as it is perceived by patients' families. The legal distinction between an act and omission in the context of treatment withdrawal is well established,[39] and crucial to establishing whether or not a medical practitioner is guilty of murder whenever they withdraw (or withhold) life-sustaining treatment. The former President of the Supreme Court has noted that categorizing switching off a life-support machine as an omission sits 'somewhat uncomfortably in terms of common sense'[40] and it is clear that in practice, when giving effect to the request requires positive steps on the part of the relevant medical professionals, the abstract legal distinction can seem very far away. As the APM guidance notes:[41]

> The withdrawal of a ventilator appears to generate more concern than withdrawing other treatments, for example fluids, in people with advanced disease. This may be because it requires a specific act that will result in death soon after. Although the death is due to the MND it can feel that the removal of a treatment caused the death and the often short time period between treatment discontinuation and death can be challenging for all concerned. The feelings engendered by the deliberate planning of a time to withdraw treatment and thus death are magnified by concerns about being seen erroneously to be assisting dying.

It is not surprising, therefore, that the GMC[42] allows a doctor to withdraw from providing care if their religious, moral, or other personal beliefs about providing life-prolonging treatment lead them to object to complying with such requests, so long as arrangements have been made for others to take over the care of the patient.

While it is unlikely that the act/omission distinction in law is going to disappear in the short- (or even medium-) term, the case study of ventilator refusal highlights just how it can break down in practice. Moreover, in practical terms, recognizing and planning for the complexities of the emotional reactions among professionals that acting on a request to withdraw treatment may well engender is an important task for senior clinicians in the ICU.

Advance refusal of treatment

Although the topic of decision making in the context of those lacking capacity is covered in greater detail in Chapter 5, advance decisions to refuse treatment

('ADRTs') merit consideration in this chapter because of the—further—challenge that they pose to the concept of the autonomous patient created by the law.

ADRTs are based on a deceptively simple idea: precedent autonomy. In other words, we should be able to project ourselves forward to a point in time when we are unable to make a decision whether to consent to or refuse a particular treatment or treatments, and that we should be able, in advance, to bind our 'incapacitated' self to the decision that we take now as to whether to refuse that treatment or treatments. As Charles J noted in *Briggs v Briggs*,[43] precedent autonomy is 'baked into' the MCA 2005 in other ways, including through the weight that decision makers acting on a best interests basis are required to place on advance written statements made when the person had capacity[44] and the ability to appoint a power of attorney with the authority to consent to or refuse medical treatment, including life-sustaining treatment.[45]

ADRTs, however, represent on the face of it the strongest form of this precedent autonomy: if the person has made an ADRT that is valid and applies to the treatment in question, then, at the point where the question arises as to whether the treatment should be given and the person lacks capacity to consent, it is as if the patient is standing before the doctor and refusing. Treatment in the face of an ADRT (if the doctor is aware of the ADRT) will give rise to criminal and civil liability,[46] and in at least one (settled) case, substantial damages have flowed from such treatment.[47] Conversely, the doctor will not face any liability for the consequences of withdrawing or withholding treatment on the basis of the ADRT.[48]

ADRTs, which were developed as common law before being put onto a statutory footing,[49] raise deep philosophical questions about the nature of personhood.[50] What is not often noticed is that their wording contains the potential for a clash between the person's past and present wishes and feelings. When the Law Commission proposed putting them on a statutory footing in the 1990s, they limited the ability of a person to 'undo' them so that they related to the circumstances when they had (when they had capacity to do so) withdrawn or altered them.[51] Section 25(2)(c) MCA 2005, as enacted, included not only such a provision but also the somewhat cryptic provision that an ADRT would cease to be valid when a person 'has done anything [...] clearly inconsistent with the advance decision remaining his fixed decision'. The word 'do' in section 25(2)(c) is pregnant with possibilities: does it mean that the person can undo the validity of their advance decision only by 'doing' something at a point when they have the capacity to realize that they are so doing, or does it mean that a person can undo an ADRT by seeking—or even accepting—medical treatment even after the point when they have lost capacity to decide whether to accept or refuse it? In other words, could the person's present, incapacitous wishes and feelings as regards medical treatment trump their prior capacitous refusal as recorded in the ADRT?

Perhaps surprisingly, given that the MCA 2005 has now been in force for over 10 years, we do not yet have a definitive answer to this question, although a passing comment in one judgment suggests that it is possible for a person to 'undo' an ADRT even from the other side of incapacity.[52] Until and unless a definitive answer is given, the strong suspicion must remain that ADRTs are only likely to constitute effective refusals of treatment when there is congruence between the clinicians, the person's family and how the person is presenting at the point when the decision has to be made. Indeed, one might well argue that, ethically, it would be unconscionable to allow treatment to be withdrawn from a person on the strength of an ADRT in the face of their (incapacitous) indication that they wanted treatment—even if the law, in most cases, does appear to direct doctors down this route.[53]

Demanding treatment

The principles

The legal principles here are clear, and summarized thus by Lady Hale in *Aintree v James*:

> A patient cannot order a doctor to give a particular form of treatment, although he may refuse it. [. . .] (para 14). In *Re J (A Minor) (Child in Care: Medical Treatment) [1991] Fam 33 at 48*, Lord Donaldson MR held that the court could not 'require the [health] authority to follow a particular course of treatment. What the court can do [in the context of a child unable to give/refuse consent on its own behalf] is to withhold consent to treatment of which it disapproves and it can express its approval of other treatment proposed by the authority and its doctors.' He repeated that view in *Re J (A Minor)(Child in Care: Medical Treatment)* [1993] Fam 15 at 26–27, when it was clearly the ratio decidendi of the case. To similar effect is *R v Cambridge District Health Authority*, ex p B [1995] 1 WLR 898, where the court would not interfere with the health authority's decision to refuse to fund further treatment of a child with leukaemia. More recently, in *R (Burke) v General Medical Council* [2005] EWCA Civ 1003, [2006] QB 273, Lord Phillips MR accepted the proposition of the General Medical Council that if a doctor concludes that the treatment which a patient wants is 'not clinically indicated he is not required (i.e., he is under no legal obligation) to provide it' (para 50), and 'Ultimately, however, a patient cannot demand

that a doctor administer a treatment which the doctor considers is adverse to the patient's clinical needs' (para 55).[54]

As discussed further in Chapter 4, these principles are now routinely challenged in the context of children by parents seeking treatment that doctors consider to be entirely futile. While none of these challenges have to date succeeded, it is likely that they will continue to be brought (often fuelled by social media and/or others jumping onto bandwagons). What is perhaps striking is that, to date, this has not applied in the context of adults. There are (infrequent) judicial review challenges to refusals to fund treatments,[55] but no cases of which we are aware whereby an adult patient has sought to challenge a decision by a doctor to refuse treatment on the basis of the doctor's assessment as to its clinical inefficacy.[56] Is this because the legal principles are so clear, or, as we explore in this section, because there is an awareness among patients of societal and resource factors, or because of the importance and power of the second opinion in the ICU context as a way of resolving any dispute?

Are some demands more 'acceptable' than others?

Decisions not to provide treatments are made because the clinician believes that the patient would not benefit from it, or because the decision has been made at a population level that that treatment cannot be funded. In the latter case, the National Institute for Health and Care Excellence regularly weighs up evidence on the safety, efficacy, and value for money of new and alternative treatments.[57] There have been examples of these decisions being challenged, for example in that of Trastuzumab (Herceptin) for breast cancer. In this case, individual patients took the relevant trusts to court, and had the decision to withhold the treatment overturned.[58]

Outside national decisions about funding such forms of treatment, however, legal cases surrounding demands for treatment are rare. That is not to say that patients demanding treatments that the doctor thinks are not in their interests is rare: quite the contrary. Patients frequently go to GPs requesting antibiotics,[59] which GPs refuse both because they do not think they would benefit the patient and also because they have a societal duty to prevent antibiotic resistance. Patients sometimes request attempted CPR even when a doctor does not believe the patient would survive such an attempt. This is such a common occurrence that the guidance from the Resuscitation Council (UK), the British Medical Association and the Royal College of Nursing has a specific section entitled 'Requests for CPR in situations where it will not be successful.[60] This recommends that such conversations ' . . . should be under-taken by clinicians with the relevant training and expertise, both in assessing the likely outcome and appropriateness of CPR, and with the relevant com-munication skills. If the patient does not accept the decision a second opinion should be offered, whenever possible.' This comment that a second opinion should be sought has its roots in both legal and clinical practice. In *R (Tracey) v Cambridge University Hospital NHS Foundation Trust and others* (covered in more detail in Chapter 3),[61] this guidance was referenced and the following was noted at paragraph 62:

> Reference has been made to Burke where Lord Phillips endorsed a number of propositions including at para 50 (v) that, if the doctor concludes that the form of treatment requested by the patient is not clinically indicated, he is under no legal obligation to provide it to the patient 'although he should offer to arrange a second opinion'. It is not clear whether Lord Phillips meant that the doctor is under a legal obligation to offer to arrange a second opinion or whether he should do so as a matter of good practice.

Quite apart from any legal directive, clinicians are happy to seek a second opinion when there is any discord between their views and that of the patient, and often even when no such discord exists. Predicting outcomes or response to treatment is a notoriously uncertain field, and it is rare to find a situation where one can predict with absolute confidence that a particular outcome will occur. It is therefore reassuring for clinicians to seek the views of their colleagues, which is often done on an informal basis but can be formalized where patients request it. Where there is concordance among clinicians that a particular outcome is likely—more suffering and eventual death for a patient in multi-organ failure on an ICU, for example—then patients are often com-fortable accepting the unanimous clinical view of futility and stop requesting treatments. The strength of the second opinion is, in our view, probably why so few cases go to court.

The same factors also hold in relation to situations where patients lack cap-acity. However, in the case of those lacking capacity, an additional complica-tion is that decisions are often formulated by clinicians on the basis that giving (or continuing) the treatment is not in the patient's best interests. As *Aintree University NHS Trust v James*[62] (covered in more detail in Chapter 5) makes clear, formulating decisions on this basis—where there is a breakdown in re-lations with the family—leaves open the door to a conclusion being reached by the court that, in fact, the treatment is in the patient's best interests.[63] This can leave the doctor in a position of doing something they feel is morally objectionable: there has not yet been a case (to our knowledge) of conscientious objection to giving a life-extending treatment said to be in the patient's best interests, but we can envisage such a situation arising.

Are some demands less acceptable than others?

One form of demand is legally unacceptable, no matter how autonomous the patient making it (applying the tests described above): a request for assistance in ending life. Section 2(1) Suicide Act[64] states: 'A person who aids, abets, counsels or procures the suicide of another, or an attempt by another to commit suicide, shall be liable on conviction on indictment to imprisonment for a term not exceeding fourteen years.'

Further, a factor in favour of prosecution under the Crown Prosecution Service guidelines[65] is that 'The suspect was acting in his or her capacity as a medical doctor, nurse, other healthcare professional, a professional carer (whether for payment or not).'

As discussed above, a refusal of life-saving treatment may, in reality, feel to the doctors concerned like a request for assistance with dying, but there is—in the eyes of the law—a clear distinction between acting on such a request and 'introducing an external agency of death.'[66] There have been repeated challenges to the Suicide Act,[67] but whatever the ethical arguments in favour of allowing defined cohorts of individuals to be given assistance to control the time and manner of their death, Parliament and the courts have to date set their face against them in contrast to—for instance—the position in Canada.[68]

Outside this clearly defined area, it seems to us that clinicians regard it as less acceptable for a patient to demand a treatment that is resource heavy and clearly might cause the patient harm: for example, surgical removal of a tumour that the surgeons stated was inoperable. More acceptable is the demand for an investigation to exclude a dangerous pathology: the anxious patient with a headache who wants to make sure they do not have a brain tumour. In this case, the risk to the patient is small (some radiation), the risk to the clinician in not doing it is great (potential litigation if the cancer gets missed), and the resource implication is sufficiently abstract that the demand is (anecdotally) often met.

The issue of resources warrants closer inspection. In areas where there is a physical limitation on resources—a countable, integer-labelled finite resource—people are happy to accept that part of the role of a healthcare system is to establish the best use of that resource. Not only can we not find a legal case of someone demanding an organ transplant, we cannot find a media story about one being demanded. Societally, we seem to be happy to accept that organs go to those who have most chance of benefiting from them, and we suppress our individual desires. In a similar vein, patients rarely request blood transfusions.

When we move one degree of abstraction away—to an ICU bed, which is countable and integer-labelled, but not necessarily finite—doctors are less happy to even reference that (part of) the reason for refusal is that the resource might be used with more efficacy elsewhere. Resources have been prayed in aid—delicately—by the Faculty of Intensive Care Medicine and the Intensive Care Society in their interventions before the Supreme Court,[69] but are rarely raised in the face-to-face interactions with individual patients. Of course, the primary reason is lack of efficacy and risk of harm to that individual, but it is disingenuous not to acknowledge that resource distribution is also a factor. Nevertheless, we wonder whether this (more abstracted) finite resource does play a role in making a demand less acceptable. It is rare (we cannot find an example in case law) for a patient to demand admission to ICU for prolonged ventilation as their lungs deteriorate. The argument for not ventilating such patients is that they would never be able to breath independently again because they have a progressive illness, but the counter-argument—for a 'demanding' patient—might be that they do not care if they never come off a ventilator, so long as they are able to (for example) see their grandchild reach its first birthday. It would, in reality, be very difficult to reject this autonomous decision on any grounds other than resource.

Conclusion

On the ICU, where literally every heartbeat is monitored and accounted for, it is very easy for doctors and patients to become focused on the moment. Doctors, having invested hours in the careful control of a patient's blood pressure and kidney function, may find it hard to remember to step back and look at the long-term prognosis for that patient: this is why it is sometimes useful for there to be a rotation of doctors, and a trigger to regularly consider best- and worst-case scenarios. Patients and relatives, in an alien environment and often sleep-deprived, may find it hard to challenge the treatment decisions being made. To ensure that good decisions are made for patients with critical illnesses, it is helpful if wishes are talked about early, conversations among doctors and those close to the patient happen regularly, and lines of communication are kept open. In these situations, and following these routes, it is unlikely that doctors will face patients 'demanding' or 'refusing' treatments, but rather will make decisions together.

References

1. Shmueli A, Sprung CL. (2005). Assessing the in-hospital survival benefits of intensive care. *Int J Technol Assess Health Care*, **21**(1), 66–72.
2. Wade DM, et al. (2012). Investigating risk factors for psychological morbidity three months after intensive care: a prospective cohort study. *Critical Care*, **16**(5), R192.
3. 'First, do no harm'.
4. http://www.healthtalk.org/peoples-experiences/intensive-care/intensive-care-experiences-family-friends/topics (accessed 20 November 2019).
5. http://icusteps.org/assets/files/IntensiveCareGuide.pdf (accessed 20 November 2019).
6. Wilson ME, et al. (2015). A video to improve patient and surrogate understanding of cardiopulmonary resuscitation choices in the ICU: a randomized controlled trial. *Crit Care Med*, **43**(3), 621–9.
7. Periyakoil VS, et al. (2014). Do unto others: doctors' personal end-of-life resuscitation preferences and their attitudes toward advance directives. *PLoS One*, **9**(5), e98246.
8. Spiegelhalter DJ. (2008). Understanding uncertainty. *Annals of Family Medicine*, **6**, 196–97.
9. *Montgomery v Lanarkshire Health Board* (Scotland) [2015] UKSC 11 at paragraph 87.
10. Resuscitation Council (UK). ReSPECT: recommended summary plan for emergency care and treatment. http://www.respectprocess.org.uk (accessed 20 November 2019), and Fritz Z, Slowther A-M, Perkins DG. (2017). Resuscitation policy should focus on the patient, not the decision. *BMJ*, **356**, j813.
11. Hoppe N, Miola J. (2014). *Medical law and medical ethics*. Cambridge University Press, Cambridge.
12. https://www.gmc-uk.org/ethical-guidance/ethical-guidance-for-doctors/good-medical-practice (accessed 20 November 2019).
13. Martin Luther King said: 'Law and order exist for the purpose of establishing justice and when they fail in this purpose they become the dangerously structured dams that block the flow of social progress.'
14. *Winspear v City Hospitals Sunderland NHS FT* [2015] EWHC 3250 (QB).
15. Bassford CR, Slowther AM, Rees K, Krucien N, Fritz Z, Quinton S, White C, Symons S, Perkins GD, Griffiths F, Dale J. (2015). *Gatekeeping in intensive*

care: understanding and improving the decision-making process surrounding ad-mission to the intensive care unit. University of Warwick, Coventry.

16. A principle first established in English law (drawing on American precedent) in *Sidaway v Board of Governors of the Bethlem Royal Hospital and Maudsley Hospital* [1985] AC 871; see also *Re T (Adult: Refusal of Medical Treatment)* [1992] 4 All ER 649.

17. *Re B* [2002] 2 All ER 449.

18. *Re B* at paragraph 100.

19. [2015] EWCOP 80; [2016] COPLR 50.

20. *Re T (Adult: Refusal of Medical Treatment)* [1992] 4 All ER 649 at 661h.

21. Section 2(4) MCA 2005.

22. *Re C* at paragraphs 29–30.

23. *Heart of England NHS Foundation Trust v JB* [2014] EWHC 342 (COP) at [7].

24. See Beauchamp TL, Childress JF. (2013). *Principles of biomedical ethics.* Oxford University Press, Oxford.

25. Kong, C. (2017). *Mental capacity in relationship: decision-making, dialogue, and autonomy.* Cambridge University Press, Cambridge.

26. See by analogy: Beaudry J-S. (2018). The way forward for medical aid in dying: pro-tecting deliberative autonomy is not enough. *Supreme Court Law Review,* second series, volume 85.

27. See further in this regard the work being done under the umbrella of the Wellcome Trust-funded Mental Health and Justice project on contested capacity assess-ment: www.mhj.org.uk (accessed 20 November 2019).

28. *Re T* at 113D.

29. *Nottinghamshire Healthcare NHS Trust v RC* [2014] EWCOP 1317 at paragraph 34.

30. *Wye Valley NHS Trust v B* [2015] EWCOP 60.

31. Ibid. at [37]. It is perhaps of note that Peter Jackson observed that this (and other state-ments) were said 'with great seriousness, and in saying it [the man] did not appear to be showing florid psychiatric symptoms or to be unduly affected by toxic infection.'

32. *Re T* at 113F-114A, 116C and 119H-120C.

33. *City of York Council v C* [2013] EWCA Civ 478; [2014] Fam 10.

34. *Re L (Vulnerable Adults with Capacity: Court's Jurisdiction)* [2012] EWCA Civ 253; [2013] Fam 1. See also *JK v A Local Health Board* [2019] EWHC 67 (Fam) for a consideration of the inherent jurisdiction in the context of medical treatment (in that case the force-feeding of a prisoner with mental health difficulties).

35. Kong, *Mental capacity in relationship.*

36. *R (Nicklinson) v Ministry of Justice* [2014] UKSC 38

37. Ibid. at paragraph 228.

38. Kong, *Mental capacity in relationship.*

39. Following *Airedale NHS Trust v Bland* [1993] AC 789.

40. *Nicklinson* at [95].
41. Kong, *Mental capacity in relationship*.
42. General Medical Council. Treatment and care towards the end of life: good practice in decision making (2010), paragraph 79.
43. *Briggs v Briggs* [2016] EWCOP 53.
44. Section 4(6)(a) MCA 2005.
45. Sections 9 and 11(8) MCA 2005.
46. Sections 26(1)-(2) MCA 2005.
47. The case of Brenda Grant, in which clinically assisted nutrition and hydration were continued for 22 months when an ADRT directing to the contrary had been misfiled. Her family received £45,000 (in an agreed settlement) in damages in consequence. See https://www.bbc.co.uk/news/uk-england-coventry-warwickshire-42240148 (accessed 20 November 2019).
48. Section 26(3) MCA 2005.
49. See, in particular, *Re AK (Adult Patient) (Medical Treatment: Consent)* [2001] 1 FLR 129 and *HE v A Hospital NHS Trust* [2003] 2 FLR 408.
50. See, for example, Law Commission (1995). *Mental incapacity* (Law Commission No 231). HMSO, London. A useful summary of the debates around Dworkin's arguments can be found in Donnelly R. (2010). *Healthcare decision-making and the law*. Cambridge University Press, Cambridge, Chapter 5.
51. Law Commission, *Mental incapacity*, paragraph 5.32.
52. *Re QQ* [2016] EWCOP 22 at [4]. Keehan J accepted that, having found that the woman in question had not had the capacity to make a valid ADRT, that even had she had capacity 'the contrary views that QQ has recently and fleetingly expressed from time to time, namely that she would accept treatment, would not of themselves invalidate, pursuant to s25 ss2 (c) of the Mental Capacity Act 2005, what would otherwise have been a valid advance decision.' In other words, he left open the possibility that more than 'fleeting' views (without capacity) might have sufficed to invalidate the decision. See also, by analogy, the discussion of the concept of advance consent to what would otherwise constitute a deprivation of liberty in Law Commission (2017). *Mental Capacity and Deprivation of Liberty* (Law Commission No 372). HMSO, London, paragraph 15.13.
53. See further Ruck Keene A, Auckland C. (2015). More presumptions please? Wishes, feelings and best interests decision-making. *Eld LJ*, 293–301.
54. *Aintree University Hospitals NHS Foundation Trust v James* [2013] UKSC 67 at paragraph 18.
55. See, for instance, *R (Rogers) v Swindon NHS Primary Care Trust* [2006] EWCA Civ 392 and *R (Condliff) v North Staffordshire PCT* [2011] EWCA Civ 910.
56. There have been challenges where a person has sought to bring such a challenge on behalf of an incapacitated adult: see, for example, *AVS v A NHS Foundation*

Trust & Anor [2011] EWCA Civ 7 (experimental treatment for Creutzfeldt-Jakob's disease).

57. See https://www.nice.org.uk (accessed 20 November 2019) for examples of their reviews.

58. *R (Rogers) v Swindon NHS Primary Care Trust* [2006] EWCA Civ 392.

59. McKay R, et al. (2016). Systematic review of factors associated with antibiotic prescribing for respiratory tract infections. *Antimicrob Agents Chemother*, **60**(7), 4106–18.

60. Decisions relating to cardiopulmonary resuscitation, 3rd edition (1st revision), 2016.

61. *R (Tracey) v Cambridge University Hospital NHS Foundation Trust and others* [2014] EWCA Civ 822.

62. *Aintree University Hospitals Trust v James* [2013] UKSC 67.

63. Another—analogous—example is *B v D* [2017] EWCOP 5, where, on the application by the person's mother, Baker J provisionally authorized the spending of funds belonging to a soldier with severe brain injuries on travel to and treatment at a clinic in Serbia with highly experimental stem cell therapy. See also the case of *University Hospitals Birmingham NHS Foundation Trust v HB* [2018] EWCOP 39, in which Keehan J considered that it was plain "that administering CPR in the event of a further collapse and giving her, albeit a very, very small chance of life, is what [the patient] would wish," such that he considered it was, at that stage, in her best interests for it to be provided to her (see paragraph 36).

64. Suicide Act 1961 section 2(1).

65. https://www.cps.gov.uk/legal-guidance/suicide-policy-prosecutors-respect-cases-encouraging-or-assisting-suicide (accessed 20 November 2019).

66. In the emotive phrase used in *Airedale NHS Trust*.

67. Most importantly, *R (Nicklinson and another) v Ministry of Justice* [2014] UKSC 38. and *R (Conway) v The Secretary of State for Justice & Ors* [2018] EWCA Civ 1431.

68. Following the ruling of the Supreme Court of Canada in *Carter v Canada* [2015] 1 SCR 331 declaring the ban on medical assistance in dying in the Canadian Criminal Code unconstitutional.

69. In *Aintree University Hospitals NHS Foundation Trust v James* [2013] UKSC 67 and *An NHS Trust v Y* [2018] UKSC 46. In Mr James's case, he had been in the ICU for 6 months by the time that the case was considered, at a very considerable cost per day (and opportunity cost in terms of the consequences for other patients), but the treating team did not advance the case that treatment should not be continued on the utilitarian ground that it was simply not cost-effective—rather they did so on the basis that such was not in his best interests.

3

DNAR: To Resuscitate or Not to Resuscitate?

Rights, Wrongs, Ethics, and the Voice of the Patient

Hazel Biggs

Introduction

Cardiopulmonary resuscitation (CPR) has been used to try to restart the heart following cardiac arrest since the 1960s. It was initially described as 'closed chest massage'[1] and since its introduction has become a commonplace procedure in healthcare settings across the UK and most other countries with developed medical care. The procedure is widely regarded as an emergency intervention conducted in circumstances where cardiac arrest was not expected and is potentially reversible. Success rates for CPR are poor, particularly if it is attempted away from hospital and by lay people, and survival to be discharged from hospital is as low as 8–10%.[2] Attempts within hospital are thought to be successful in only 15–20% of cases.[3] Performing CPR often involves the risk of harm associated with the procedures involved, or because it may exacerbate the patient's underlying condition, or further prolong and aggravate the dying process.

At its most basic, CPR tends to be limited to forceful manual compressions of the chest to stimulate cardiac function and encourage the circulation of oxygenated blood to the brain and heart. However, in hospital settings like the intensive care unit (ICU), it usually also involves ventilation of the lungs and the use of a range of equipment. At a minimum, pocket masks and oral airways may be used, but more invasive and complex interventions would include laryngeal mask airways, self-inflating bags, and tracheal intubation. Drugs are typically administered to help stimulate cardiac output and circulation, and electrical defibrillation is also commonplace in hospitals and increasingly in the community.

Chest compressions and defibrillation have been regarded by some as 'a desperate measure that involves somewhat brutal force to revive a non-pulsating heart'[4] and have become one of the more contentious aspects of CPR. Indeed, in frail elderly patients, CPR has been described as a 'violent and undignified' technique,[5] and in critical or intensive care, where the patient's prospects of survival may already be severely compromised, the possibility of causing injury through strenuous CPR will be a significant factor in clinical decisions about whether or not to attempt resuscitation. 'Do not attempt resuscitation (DNAR)' decisions have therefore proven ethically and legally contentious, and there is also some research that shows that the implementation of such decisions can sometimes be practically and ethically misunderstood.[6] For patients, the potential use of CPR may be a welcome intervention that could prolong life, or it might be a prospect that they wish to avoid, particularly in instances where this violent intervention is regarded as undignified and potentially futile. The legal and ethical landscape associated with the administration of CPR will be considered in this chapter, including an assessment of the position where the patient disagrees with a DNAR order, the implications of resuscitation without consent, DNAR decisions in the context of their practical application, and some analysis of the potential liability for failure to resuscitate.

'Do not attempt resuscitation' decisions

In the public consciousness, resuscitation is often mistakenly regarded as a life-saving procedure, about which many have unrealistic expectations about the likely success and benefits. Research has shown that CPR is erroneously thought to be successful in 50% of cases.[7] False perceptions and inflated ideas as to the likelihood of success are often fuelled by dramatic media depictions of successful outcomes, which tend to gloss over the realities of the process of resuscitation.[8]

Consequently, a decision not to attempt resuscitation is often perceived as a harbinger of imminent death, particularly in the environment of the ICU. In such situations, it may be difficult for patients and their loved ones to accept a clinical decision that seems unnecessarily final, so that these decisions are frequently contentious and can result in misunderstandings and loss of trust between doctor and patient. Nevertheless, good clinical practice dictates that such decisions must be made even though they are inevitably fraught with ambiguity and often imprecision.

It is a truism that everybody who dies suffers a cardiac arrest: it is the ultimate clinical sign of death. Sometimes, therefore, cardiac arrest simply represents the natural end to life, particularly when associated with the end stages of terminal illness. To subject a patient to an invasive and potentially harmful medical intervention such as CPR in these circumstances, where a successful outcome is unlikely and unrealistic, would be contrary to their best interests (or, in Scotland, without overall benefit) and clinically inappropriate. Performing CPR when quality of life after the procedure would inevitably be diminished offends the ethical principle of non-maleficence. It would also almost certainly be unlawful, because treatment should only be administered if it is demonstrably in the patient's best interests.

Consequently, it has been argued that 'It is appropriate to consider making a DNR order when attempted CPR will almost certainly not restart the patient's heart, when there is no benefit in so doing or when the expected benefits are outweighed by the burdens.'[9] However, despite the apparent clarity of this statement, a patient faced with a choice of whether or not to accept CPR might, at a minimum, be expected to question the meaning of 'almost certainly' before agreeing to a DNAR decision. They might also be interested in how accurately the prospective benefits and burdens can be assessed in order to determine which was the most significant. For instance, is CPR expected to be of no benefit because it is unlikely to succeed in any event, or because the prognosis is very poor and successful resuscitation would simply prolong the dying process? Or, would it be that the burdens of painful and distressing potential side effects of CPR, such as severe bruising and fractured ribs or sternum, clearly outweigh any possible benefits because the patient is already frail. Ordinarily, a clinical decision that a specific treatment option or intervention would be contrary to a patient's best interests would mean that a clinician is not obliged to offer that treatment and the patient would not necessarily be informed about it as a treatment option, but the position is more complex in relation to CPR.

Clinically, the potential burdens of providing CPR relate both to the nature of the intervention and the quality of life the patient will be likely to enjoy afterwards. A number of factors, including age, terminal illness, cancer, sepsis, pneumonia, and renal failure, among others, are known to have a detrimental influence on the outcome of CPR. As a consequence, CPR is usually regarded as inappropriate in patients with these conditions, except in rare cases where the cardiac crisis results from a temporary and readily reversible cause such as choking or a blocked tracheostomy tube.[10] Further, if the coronary failure is directly related to the disease process, then successful resuscitation will often achieve nothing more than simply prolonging the dying process. In these cases, when it is unlikely that performing CPR will enhance, or even maintain the patient's quality of life, it will not be regarded as in the patient's best interests and a DNAR order will usually be appropriate. In other patients, the prognosis following CPR may be more optimistic and here the decision about whether and when it will be appropriate to resuscitate turns on a number of factors.

Both medical ethics and law dictate that calculating a patient's best interests involves social and welfare concerns as well as the purely medical,[11] implying that quality of life measures are as important as quantity of life. Best interests is also central to the decision-making process because the doctor has a duty to treat the patient according to their best interests. Hence, in end of life decision making, a best interests analysis is pivotal to the determination of what treatment options to offer.

It has long been the legal position, based on sound moral and ethical principles such as beneficence and non-maleficence, that there is no requirement to 'strive officiously' to keep a patient alive when to do so would be futile.[12] Furthermore, even some of the major religions have accepted that CPR represents extraordinary treatment that will not benefit every patient, thereby recognizing that quality of life may override sanctity of life in some cases.[13] Despite this, deciding not to treat based on an assessment of an individual's quality of life has always been controversial, especially when the patient is unable to decide for themselves, as in the American case of Clare Conroy: 'We do not believe that it would be appropriate for a court to designate a person with authority to determine that someone else's life is not worth living simply because, to that person, the patient's "quality of life" or value to society seems negligible.'[14]

The courts of England and Wales have, however, confirmed that it is lawful to withhold CPR from a patient who lacks decision-making capacity when it would be contrary to their best interests.[15] But, in relation to a DNACPR decision, determining the patient's best interests is complex, and these decisions are particularly controversial given the expectations that it is a life-preserving treatment.[16] The facts of the case of *Tracey v Cambridge University Hospital Trust* epitomize the depth of feeling that can be generated in circumstances such as this.

Mrs Tracey was admitted to Addenbrooke's Hospital, Cambridge, having suffered fractures to her cervical spine in a road traffic accident. Two weeks prior to the accident, she had been diagnosed with terminal lung cancer, with a life expectancy of approximately nine months. On admission, she also had a chest infection and her respiration was impaired, so she was placed on a ventilator. After a week, her case was reviewed and it was decided to remove the ventilator. The treating anaesthetist in intensive care then completed a DNAR order (cited in the case as the first order). This order was later revoked after Mrs Tracey's family became aware of it and protested that it had been applied without consultation with the patient or her family at a time when Mrs Tracey had expressed a wish 'to receive full active treatment'.[17] Mrs Tracey's condition improved briefly, and during this period she wrote a note during a medical consultation about her future care, stating 'please do not exclude me'.[18] Sadly, her condition later deteriorated significantly, and a second DNAR order was made with the agreement of her family. She subsequently died.

After Mrs Tracey's death, her family brought a claim against the hospital trust in relation to the first DNAR order. They claimed that Mrs Tracey's right to a private and family life under Article 8 of the European Convention on Human Rights (ECHR) had been breached when the trust failed to consult with the patient or her family before imposing the DNAR order. Further, they complained that there had been no notification that the order had been made, and there had been no offer of a second opinion. It was also argued that the trust's DNARCPR policy was not made available to Mrs Tracey and that the trust had failed to have a policy that was 'clear and unambiguous'. An additional claim was brought against the Secretary of State, who was alleged to have breached Mrs Tracey's Article 8 rights for failing to publish national guidance ensuring that 'the process for making DNARCPR orders is sufficiently clear, accessible and foreseeable'. It was argued that people like Mrs Tracey have a right to be involved in the DNARCPR decision-making process and given appropriate information to allow them meaningful involvement, including the right to seek a second opinion.[19]

These claims are founded on concerns for the autonomy, integrity, dignity and quality of life of the patient under the Article 8 right to protect one's private life, which reflects ethical principles associated with medical decision making.[20, 21] However, the counter arguments in *Tracey* raised concerns as to whether failure to consult on a DNACPR order could in fact engage this particular right. Relying on the earlier case of *Tysiac v Poland*[22] in the European Court of Human Rights, the court concluded that Article 8 was engaged, stating that 'private life is a broad term, encompassing, inter alia, aspects of an individual's physical and social identity, including personal autonomy'.[23] Furthermore, in line with *Tysiac*, it was argued that the Convention is designed to uphold real rights, 'not rights that are theoretical or illusory, but rights that are practical and effective'.[24, 25] *Tracey* also confirmed at paragraph 29 that:

[W]hat has to be determined is whether, having regard to the particular circumstances of the case and notably the nature of the decisions to be taken, an individual has been involved in the decision-making process, seen as a whole, to a degree sufficient to provide her or him with the requisite protection of their interests.[26]

In light of this, it was argued in *Tracey* that 'A decision as to how to pass the closing days and moments of one's life and how one manages one's death touches in the most immediate and obvious way a patient's personal autonomy, integrity, dignity and quality of life',[27] which is at the heart of the Article 8 right to a private and personal life.

The court found that there should always be 'a presumption in favour of patient involvement' in DNACPR decision making[28] unless to do so would cause physical or psychological harm. That is not to say, however, that discussion can be avoided if it is thought that the patient might find it distressing. The court was emphatic that these decisions are of a different order to everyday treatment decisions. And, even though a clinician cannot be compelled to provide treatment that is believed to be contrary to the patient's best interests, failing to discuss the issue of resuscitation, or make the patient aware that an order is in place, breaches the patient's rights and deprives them of the opportunity to seek a second opinion.[29]

Ultimately, the claims of the Tracey family were upheld and a declaration was granted against the hospital trust, such that by failing to involve Mrs Tracey in the decision-making process it had violated her right to respect for private life under Article 8. In the context of DNAR, *Tracey* confirmed many previous judgments that respect for patient autonomy is paramount in decision making. The later case of *Winspear v City Hospitals Sunderland NHS Foundation Trust*, which concerned a failure to consult the carer of a mentally incapacitated adult before imposing a DNARCPR order, reiterated the fact that inconvenience and concerns about difficult conversations do not negate this right.[30] With regard to the ability to access a second opinion, however, the court stopped short of finding that there was a *legal* obligation to offer a second opinion about DNAR decisions. Nevertheless, the availability of a second opinion is widely regarded as an important aspect of medical decision making, and the General Medical Council (GMC) recommends obtaining a second opinion in cases where there is disagreement about end of life care planning.[31]

The sensitivities involved in these decisions, and discussions about end of life care are well known, and the issues associated with DNAR decisions are especially problematic given the public perceptions that they are of life-saving significance. It is therefore unsurprising that, since the judgment in *Tracey*, many examples of professional and ethical guidance have been developed or updated outlining the legal and ethical imperatives associated with the DNAR orders and designed to assist clinicians in the decision-making process.

'Do not attempt cardiopulmonary resuscitation' policies

As long ago as 1991, the then chief medical officer for England advised that consultants and chief executives are responsible for ensuring that resuscitation policies are in place and understood by all staff. Since then, various policies have been published and updated, with the British Medical Association (BMA), Royal College of Nursing (RCN), and Resuscitation Council first publishing joint guidance in 2007[32] and the GMC publishing its guidance on end of life care for doctors in 2010.[33] In Scotland, comprehensive NHS guidance was published in 2010,[34] introducing a uniform policy on DNACPR policy across a full range of institutions, from hospitals and care homes to ambulance crews and the Scottish Police Force. The Scottish guidance was updated in 2016 to reflect recent case law, and offers a comprehensive and detailed policy on communication and decision making.[35] The NHS in Wales also has a DNAR policy that applies across all healthcare settings, which includes a copy of the standard form to record the decision and decision-making process.[36] In England, however, the position is less uniform, and a report by the National Confidential Enquiry into Patient Outcomes and Death (NCEPOD), entitled *Time to intervene?*, was published in 2012 responding to claims that too many physicians 'have drifted into an expectation that death will provoke a physical intervention as part of a last ditch attempt to prolong life'.[37] Inconsistencies in practice between hospitals were also highlighted, prompting the report to call for a change of approach.

Following the judgment in *Tracey* in 2014, several further publications and studies of DNAR orders indicate that there has been a shift towards formalizing the process of implementing and documenting DNACPR orders in clinical practice. The most recent and influential of these is the updated joint guidance prepared by the BMA, RCN, and Resuscitation Council in 2016.[38] This guidance reiterates and reinforces previous ethical and regulatory guidelines on good clinical practice in this area—namely, that decisions about whether or not to resuscitate should ideally be taken as part of advance care planning for any patient to whom it may be relevant, which will include many of those receiving critical or intensive care. Good end of life care should also include discussions about DNAR orders and the benefits and burdens associated with CPR, and there should be no need to involve the courts unless there is a dispute between the doctor and patient or their representatives if they are incapacitated. Ethically and legally, a DNAR order is not solely a clinical decision. It involves an assessment of the patient's best interests and quality of life, and patient autonomy requires that where possible the patient should be involved in the decision-making process.[39]

However, the ethical and professional guidance developed by the various professional bodies such as the GMC and BMA is largely advisory rather than mandatory. Consequently, individual hospital trusts in England have tended to develop local guidance based on their own experiences. It was acknowledged in the judgment in *Tracey*, however, that 'inconsistency and confusion continues to exist' over DNACPR decisions and policies, which is cause for concern.[40] The Joint Statement of 2016 recommended that written information about CPR policies should also be provided in general literature to patients and made readily available—an approach that was also endorsed by the BMA in the model patient information leaflet it developed in 2008 and updated in 2017.[41] Furthermore, to be compliant with Article 8, healthcare trusts' policies on DNACPR must be clear and accessible, as well as precise and understandable to the patient.[42] Yet, in 2015, it was noted in Parliament that 'Communication failings appear at all levels ... healthcare professionals are not always having the open and honest conversations that are necessary for carers and family members to understand both the severity of the situation and also the choices that will need to be made.'[43]

Greater consistency in DNAR decision making may be facilitated by national guidance, and the value of a national policy like the one that existed in Scotland at the time was discussed in *Tracey* in relation to the claim that the Secretary of State had neglected his duty under Article 8 of the ECHR by failing to ensure the implementation of a national policy.[44] The court decided, however, that the issues associated with poor communication around DNAR orders would not be solved by the implementation of a national policy, but were instead more influenced by the difficulties inherent in the decision-making process and attached to the sensitivities of DNACPR generally. Regardless of this, the judgment also acknowledged that inconsistencies in DNAR decisions and their application needed to be ironed out as far as possible[45] and commentators continue to call for the introduction of national guidance to ensure consistency of approach and patient safety.[46] The importance of these claims should not be underestimated, however, because it seems likely that the lack of uniform guidance may be responsible for the inconsistencies in the implementation of DNACPR policies that continue to occur in clinical practice with detrimental effects for patients.[47]

Patients are clearly being disadvantaged and potentially confused if they are not receiving clear, open, and honest information about their clinical outlooks and possible treatments, particularly in relation to end of life care. Alongside the disregard for patients' rights associated with poor communication, there is also concern that without a standard form of guidance, or a national policy to inform the process of DNAR decision making, some patients may be receiving 'suboptimal' care in practice.[48]

Clinical uncertainty and patient detriment

Alongside public misapprehensions about the implications of resuscitation, there is increasing evidence to show that misunderstandings have occurred among healthcare professionals regarding the significance and practical impact of DNAR orders. Several studies demonstrate that these misunderstandings and misinterpretations have sometimes resulted in the inappropriate withdrawal of all care from patients at the end of life.[49, 50, 51] Such misunderstandings are not limited to the UK, and have also been noted in the USA[52, 53] and various European countries.[54] In Ireland, for example, one study recently reported that '26% of staff nurses and 30% of primary care physicians surveyed' believed that patients with a DNAR order could not receive interventions from an extensive list of treatments, including antibiotics, intravenous fluids, and, astonishingly, pain relief.[55] The extent of the lack of sound understanding of the clinical implications of a DNAR order shown in this survey is very worrying. It was reported that 20% of the Irish primary care doctors surveyed thought that a patient with a DNAR could not be referred to hospital from a nursing home, and 'over one quarter of staff nurses and almost one-third of primary care physicians believe that a DNAR can preclude patients from receiving even elements of basic care.'[56]

The extent of the potential harm to patients is perhaps best illustrated by a large study of surgical patients that clearly demonstrated that patients with DNACPR orders have significantly higher morbidity in hospital than patients with similar medical conditions but no DNACPR order.[57]

Ethically and legally, patients have a right to receive appropriate clinically indicated medical care regardless of their medical condition and prognosis, but it seems that all too often that right is not upheld in practice for patients with DNAR orders. The evidence demonstrating that these patients often receive different, and detrimental, treatment compared with their peers is particularly troubling in the context of a human rights analysis, because it suggests that this group of vulnerable patients may be being systematically discriminated against. The reasons behind the misunderstandings of the effect of DNAR orders on treatment are complex, and difficult to determine with any certainty, but some authors conclude that they may be associated with the emphasis that the DNACPR order places on withholding treatment. Although the DNAR order is specific to withholding resuscitation and does not speak to other treatments, there is some suggestion that the specific weight placed on *not* treating is likely to be responsible for at least some of the misapprehensions about wider clinical care associated with them.[58]

One issue that could be influencing this relates to different understandings and applications of relevant ethical principles.[59] For instance, a recent study[60] discovered that DNACPR policies are allowed in only 71% of 31 European countries surveyed, meaning that 29% of those countries did not routinely operate DNAR policies, although this had increased significantly since an earlier study.[61] Interestingly, this study[62] also reveals that Germany has a highly developed policy on who should be involved in DNAR decision making, which is enshrined in law, unlike in the UK and most other countries. Also notable is the guide to end of life decision making drawn up by the Committee on Bioethics (DH-BIO) of the Council of Europe,[63] which was developed to try to protect the rights of patients in relation to the implementation of the principles enshrined in the Convention on Human Rights and Biomedicine.[64] Based on shared values and established ethical principles such as autonomy, beneficence, and non-maleficence, the guide provides comprehensive guidance for patients, their families, and healthcare professionals about end of life decision making and the processes involved. It is lamentable that this useful document, which places the protection of human dignity at its heart, has not been more influential in informing policy and practice.

There are still indications that patients are not receiving good information about decisions relating to their end of life care, despite their right to be involved in the decision-making process so that they are fully informed and able to exercise autonomy. Along with other ethical guidance, the Council of Europe's guide discusses the need for transparency in decision making so that patients are enabled to exercise their autonomy[65] and are not harmed by a lack of knowledge. It is possible, however, that the requirement for clarity and accessibility of information may be undermined for patients and healthcare professionals alike by the use of a wide range of different terminologies and acronyms used in local guidelines and policies, such as DNAR, DNACPR, and AND ('allow natural death') among others. In addition, the use of various different approaches to recording formalities and practice delivery can result in uncertainty and confusion for medical professionals.[66] And one consequence of this may be the conflation of DNACPR decisions with end of life care generally, which is thought to be widespread and a cause of some of the harmful practices evidenced above.[67, 68]

Since the factors to be considered for each decision about CPR are multifaceted and largely specific to each patient, it is logical that they should be made on an individual basis, putting the patient at the heart of the decision-making process. In the past, however, great controversy has been generated by blanket policies applied to specific classes of patients—for example, elderly people or those with dementia. Blanket policies clearly have discriminatory tendencies and it would therefore be unethical, and almost certainly unlawful under the Human Rights Act 1998, for healthcare institutions to implement such a policy. In the case of older people, they would also contravene the Department of Health and Social Care's *Service framework for older people.*[69] The needs and interests of each individual patient should be at the heart of policies on DNAR and end of life care generally (see reference 63) but it is clear that patients' concerns in relation to CPR tend to focus on two main aspects—namely, inappropriate resuscitation and disagreement with DNAR orders made for them. The law and ethics associated with these two areas will now be considered.

Inappropriate resuscitation

The competent patient has an absolute right to refuse treatment[70] and may exercise this right for their own personal reasons, or indeed for no reason at all.[71] Such a refusal may be made in advance using an advance decision refusing treatment as discussed in Chapter 2. The ReSPECT initiative, which stands for Recommended Summary Plan for Emergency Care and Treatment, is founded on similar principles and is of particular value for those with complex medical needs towards the end of their lives. It locates the person at the centre of decision making, with an emphasis on future care needs and advance decision making.[72] In circumstances where a patient is properly informed and counselled and yet refuses CPR, it is likely that they do so out of strongly held convictions, either because they do not wish their life to be prolonged if they suffer a cardiac arrest, or they do not wish to suffer the indignity of intensive CPR. For instance, even if there appears to be a good chance that CPR will revive the patient, other factors, such as perhaps the perceived indignity of the process or the effects on those close to them, may dictate that they regard resuscitation as undesirable and cause them to reject it. Such a patient may suffer emotional and psychological harm as a consequence of CPR performed inappropriately, and would be at liberty to bring an action for battery in relation to the resuscitation or any other physical life-saving treatment administered to them.

Nevertheless, concerns continue to be raised about inappropriate resuscitation in circumstances where success is clinically unlikely, even when the patient has not been consulted. For instance, one commentator recounted 'A memorable letter he received from the family of a patient that described resuscitation as "the routine, institutionalised electrocution and torture of the dying"'.[73] The *Tracey* case also recognized this kind of disproportionate and futile medical intervention as being problematic[74] and it has been rightly described elsewhere as 'undignified'.[75] There are clearly tensions between the expectations of patients and the use of resuscitation in clinical practice despite the wealth of ethical guidance available, and patients would be within their rights to bring a legal challenge for inappropriate resuscitation if CPR is performed against their wishes or without consultation and consent.

Having argued that ethics and law require that patients should be informed of the brutal truths about CPR and its chances of success before reaching a decision, that decision ought to be respected and the law should make amends if it is not. It is one thing to treat a patient in the absence of consent, but quite another to do so over their express refusal, especially in a life and death situation. However, should CPR succeed in these circumstances, it would seem counter-intuitive to argue that clinicians, whose primary professional imperative is to save life, should be held accountable for preserving the life of a patient. Likewise, one might expect that—morally—most of society would regard life as preferable to death, and conventional legal wisdom would suggest that the law would not construe continued life, or existence, resulting from CPR as a harm. Rather, being alive would usually be perceived as a beneficial outcome that would be unlikely to permit a patient to successfully sue for damages.[76] However, 'some people have a profound abhorrence of being kept alive in a state of total dependency or permanent lack of awareness, or of undignified death',[77] which might lead them to decide not to accept CPR if it were offered. Others may simply feel that, when their 'time has come', they would prefer to experience death without the intrusion of invasive medical procedures. In these circumstances, the imposition of CPR could represent a grave and undignified violation of personal autonomy.

There is limited UK case law on this type of issue, but is perhaps best illustrated by the case of *Ms B*[78] in what seems to be the only UK case to date to address the issue of a life being maintained against the wishes of a patient. Ms B was irreversibly paraplegic and was being maintained by mechanical respiration following complications resulting from a cavernoma in her neck. Once her diagnosis was established, she withdrew her consent to the treatment and requested that the life support system be removed. The hospital declined to do so, arguing inter alia that she was not competent to make the decision. She challenged the hospital's failure to comply with her wishes and, having ascertained that she was competent to decide for herself, the court found in her favour. In the absence of consequential harm, she was awarded nominal damages of £100 for battery in respect of the violation of her physical integrity, and the hospital was required to respect her autonomous refusal of consent and withdraw the treatment—an outcome that suggests that it would be possible to establish that a legal harm can result from CPR performed unlawfully (that is, without the patient's consent).

Compensation could be sought under various heads of claim, not just for pain and suffering in relation to the physical aspects of the treatment but also primarily for the affront to the patient's autonomy and the denial of their wishes.[79] It might be difficult to envisage that a court would find against a defendant who had acted in good faith to attempt to benefit a patient, but that is exactly what happened in a case involving the George Eliot Hospital, Nuneaton, in 2017.[80] Here, the patient, Brenda Grant, had made an advance decision to refuse treatment, making it clear that she feared loss of dignity and degradation more than she feared death, and did not want treatment to prolong her life, including artificial feeding, should she suffer one of a range of illnesses and no longer have decision-making capacity. She later suffered a catastrophic stroke, but her advance decision was misplaced among her medical records and she was artificially fed for 22 months. The family having argued that the hospital trust neglected its duty under tort law for not respecting her living will and keeping her alive against her will, the Hospital Trust settled the claim and paid the family £45,000 in damages.

Damages in tort are designed to put the claimant in the position they would occupy had the tort not occurred, as far as money can do so. Clearly, had the patient not been resuscitated, they would be dead, and no amount of money can 'restore' them to that position. One alternative would be to claim special damages, the quantum of which would be calculated according to the costs associated with their continued existence. While this might be appropriate in privately funded health care systems such as the USA, it would not be appropriate, or necessary, to claim the direct costs of medical care when treatment is provided by the National Health Service. Additional costs, such as ordinary living expenses and perhaps the costs of social care, which would have been avoided by death, might be sought, but in Re T (Adult: Refusal of Treatment)[81] the judge doubted that compensation of this type would be available, although substantial damages were awarded in the Canadian case of Malette v Shulman.[82] Malette's position seems to be supported by authorities from the

USA[83, 84] where the courts appealed to social morality as the foundation of their refusal to recognize a prolonged life as harm capable of compensation. Redress for harm caused by the denial of autonomy in relation to the actual resuscitation, as occurred in the case of Brenda Grant, is clearly the most appropriate approach rather than any injury brought about by the fact that the patient is alive against their express wishes.[85] It is, as Strasser argues, a claim born of the derogation of the right to physical integrity,[86] and as such the ordinary principles of tort law should be applied. This allows people whose valid refusal of life-saving treatment has been disregarded to succeed[87] in the same way that those who have consented to treatment, but without being fully informed of all potential consequences, can succeed. Failing to compensate in these situations would leave the patient with no remedy in circumstances where the clinician was in clear breach of a professional duty, and 'a claimant ought not to be without a remedy, even if it involves some extension of existing principle' because otherwise that duty would 'in many cases be drained of its content'.[88]

'Do not attempt resuscitation' without consent

The case of *Tracey*, discussed above, focuses on the law and ethics of DNAR decisions that are imposed without the patient's knowledge and consent. In that particular instance, the patient did not need resuscitation and the DNAR order in question was withdrawn. In different circumstances, however, the imposition of a DNR order without consent or consultation, combined with subsequent failure to provide CPR resulting in death, is perhaps the most obvious, or at least the most foreseeable, reason for a legal challenge to decision making of this type, especially if the existence of a DNAR order was not known to the patient or their relatives. Whether or not such a challenge would succeed depends on a number of factors, but is most likely to turn on whether, in the circumstances that arose, the clinician concerned was in breach of a legal obligation to provide CPR to the specific patient.

It is clear that the overriding legal duty of any doctor is to treat each patient according to their best interests. The determination of what constitutes the best interests of a specific patient depends on their medical condition, the treatment proposed, and the views and wishes of the patient, if known. In the case of adult patients lacking capacity, the medical, social, and welfare implications of providing, or not providing, the treatment should be considered under the Mental Capacity Act 2005 in England and Wales, or the Adults with Incapacity (Scotland) Act 2000. Case law has firmly established that where a clinical assessment indicates that a particular intervention, such as CPR, would be contrary to a patient's best interests, the doctor is not obliged to offer that treatment, even if the patient requests it. Specifically, where a treatment is regarded as futile or where any potential benefit is outweighed by the concomitant harms, the principle of non-maleficence dictates that it would be unethical to provide it and a clinician is under no obligation to do so.[89,90] That is settled law and ethically justifiable, but in relation to CPR, where the decision might seem to turn on a choice between certain death and the promise of survival, discord is perhaps predictable.

Some patients may not be content to accept a DNR decision, having their own 'specific reasons for wanting to try to delay death',[91] and this wish may persist even after full and frank discussion of the potential risks and benefits of CPR and the prospects of success. If in these circumstances no agreement can be reached, the clinician faces a real ethical dilemma: whether to disregard a potentially dying patient's wish, or to provide a potentially harmful treatment against clinical judgement. Confusingly, it has recently been suggested that:

> If, in spite of clinical evidence that CPR is more likely to cause harm than provide benefit, the patient still requests that CPR be attempted, that wish should normally be respected. Although the healthcare team may disagree that the risks posed by CPR are justified ... it is for the individual himself to accept that chance.[92]

Advice such as this runs counter to the law and most policy guidance, but epitomizes the kinds of clinical dilemmas that frequently occur in practice. Extra-clinical factors, including the patient's own personal and subjective understanding of their quality of life, will undoubtedly influence their decision whether or not to agree to a DNAR order. When this leads the patient to reject a proposed DNAR and accept the risks associated with the procedure, the clinician who responds as suggested above is respecting their autonomy and right to decide, while potentially compromising their best interests. In this regard, as David Price explains, 'the threshold of burdensomeness will differ from one person to another'.[93] The nature of the treatment and the decision-making process also lend themselves to the inevitability that some patients will lose their resolve and change their minds when faced with their mortality, and request resuscitation even after a DNAR has been agreed.[94, 95]

When the clinician and patient cannot agree and the patient continues to seek CPR and refuses to consent to a DNAR order, a second opinion, as considered in *Tracey*, would be a valuable intervention. If agreement still cannot be reached, the courts can be called on to adjudicate and judgment would turn on issues related to the assessment of the individual patient's best interests and draw heavily upon jurisprudence relating to medical decisions about patients who lack capacity to decide for themselves.[96] Perhaps most influential among these is *Burke*,[97] where the Court of Appeal determined conclusively that 'Autonomy and the right to self-determination do not entitle the patient to insist on receiving a particular medical treatment regardless of the nature of that treatment'.[98] Put simply, a doctor cannot be required to provide treatment, even resuscitation, against their clinical judgement,[99] but the damaging potential loss of trust and breakdown of the doctor–patient relationship that is likely to occur if a clinician holds firm to the decision to withhold CPR is undoubtedly what is driving the call above to simply respect the patient's wish. Moreover, it has been held more recently that if administering CPR is clearly what a patient would wish then it can, in some circumstances, be regarded as in their best interests for it to be performed[100] even if the clinical team disagrees.

Conclusions

The foregoing discussion makes clear that DNAR discussions are unquestionably difficult to broach, but failing to have the discussion with patients and their representatives raises concerns about communication and trust, as seen in *Tracey* and various accusatory headlines in the media.[101] The law surrounding 'do not attempt cardiopulmonary resuscitation' (DNACPR) orders is based on sound ethical principles, and patients' rights to be involved in DNACPR decisions. Nevertheless, these decisions continue to be ethically controversial, confusing for patients, and frequently poorly understood or misinterpreted by healthcare practitioners.

Discussion and communication are central to the decision-making process, and there is a great deal of evidence to suggest that most patients welcome discussion, or at least some consultation, about CPR and its relevance to them.[102] [103] Conversely, failure to discuss CPR with competent patients can lead others to make decisions that would actively be contrary to their wishes. There are then compelling arguments in favour of discussing the matter with the patient as part of their advance care planning, and prior to CPR becoming necessary, as enshrined in the ReSPECT initiative. In the past, however, some scholars have also argued that consultation on DNAR may be detrimental, even psychologically harmful to some,[104] reinforcing clinical uncertainty.

The vast array of policies relating to DNAR all support the need for good communication, emphasizing that patient autonomy should be promoted and decision making should be based on mutual discussions between healthcare professionals and patients and their carers. But this research shows that the clinical impacts of DNAR in practice are still often being misinterpreted, resulting in inappropriate withdrawal of other treatments. Some patients are also still being subjected to CPR in circumstances where it is unwelcome and burdensome. In this environment, it is unsurprising that patients and their relatives continue to be mistrustful of the process by which DNAR orders are decided upon and implemented.

Given the continuing controversy surrounding DNAR despite the legal clarity and extensive ethical and professional guidance already available, it now seems clear that a new approach is needed. Some commentators have advocated a move to the Universal form of Treatment Options (UFTO) as an alternative[105] and there is merit in this suggestion. There is evidence to indicate that the UFTO leads to better patient outcomes and a reduction of harm associated with DNAR orders, but the real issue is why DNAR orders continue to cause harmful outcomes for patients. It is now imperative that clear and consistent guidance is developed and established as mandatory across the healthcare sector to ensure that patients receive high-quality end of life care that enables them to exercise their autonomy without unnecessarily burdening them. This needs to be supported by education and training and backed up by clear policies on practical implementation and professional regulation, with potential legal sanctions attached to non-compliance and poor performance. Only then will patients' rights be upheld and their voices heard and appreciated.

References

1. Kouwenhoven WB, Jude JR, Knickerbocker GG. (1960). Closed chest cardiac massage. *J Am Med Soc*, **173**, 1064–1067.
2. Daya MR, Schmicker RH, Zive DM, et al. (2015). Resuscitation Outcomes Consortium investigators. Out of hospital cardiac arrest survival results from Resuscitation Outcomes Consortium (ROC). *Resuscitation*, **91**, 108–15.
3. Nolan JP, Soar J, Smith GB, et al. (2014). Incidence and outcome of in-hospital cardiac arrest in the United Kingdom national cardiac arrest audit. *Resuscitation*, **85**, 987–92.
4. Gelbman BD, Gelbman JM. (2008). Deconstructing DNR. *J Med Ethics*, **34**, 640–1, at 641.
5. Wilson J. (2008). To what extent should older patients be included in decisions regarding their resuscitation status? *J Med Ethics*, **34**, 353–6, at 354.
6. Stewart M. (2011). The over-interpretation of DNAR. *Clinical Governance*, **16**, 119–28.

7. Van den Bulck JJ. (2002). The impact of television fiction on public expectations of survival following inhospital cardiopulmonary resuscitation by medical professionals. *European Journal of Emergency Medicine*, **9**, 325–9.

8. Diem S, Lantos JD, Tulsky JA. (1996). Cardiopulmonary resuscitation on television: miracles and misinformation. *New England J Medicine*, **334(24)**, 1578–82.

9. Mason JK, Laurie G. (2013). *Mason & McCall-Smith's law and medical ethics*, 4th edn. Oxford University Press, Oxford.

10. British Medical Association, Resuscitation Council (UK), Royal College of Nursing (2016). *Do not attempt CPR: decisions relating to cardiopulmonary resuscitation*, 3rd edn (1st revision). https://www.resus.org.uk/dnacpr/decisions-relating-to-cpr (accessed 4 December 2019).

11. *Re A (Male Sterilisation)* [2000] 1 FLR 549, at 556.

12. Bayliss R. (1982). Thou shalt not strive officiously. **285**, 1373–5.

13. Pius XII: The prolongation of life (1958). *The Pope Speaks*, **4**, as cited by Saunders J. (1996). Medical futility: CPR. In: Lee R, Morgan D, eds, *Death rites: law and ethics at the end of life*. Routledge, London, at 76.

14. *Re Clare Conroy* 486 A 2d 1209 (NJ. 1985).

15. *Re R (Adult: Medical Treatment)* [1996] 2 FLR 99.

16. *Tracey v Cambridge Uni Hospital Trust* [2014] EWCA Civ 822.

17. *Tracey*, at para 11.

18. *Tracey*, at para 13.

19. *Tracey*, at para 7.

20. *Pretty v Director of Public Prosecutions* [2001] UKHL 61.

21. *Tracey*, at para 32.

22. *Tysiac v Poland* (2007) 45 ECHR 42.

23. *Tysiac*, at para 109.

24. *Tysiac*, at para 115.

25. *Tracey*, at para 37.

26. *Tysiac*, at para 115.

27. *Tracey*, at para 32.

28. *Tracey*, at para 53.

29. *Tracey*, at para 55.

30. *Winspear v City Hospitals Sunderland NHS Foundation Trust* [2015] EWHC 3250.

31. General Medical Council (2010). *Treatment and care towards the end of life: good practice in decision making*, General Medical Council, London, at para 47.

32. British Medical Association, Royal College of Nursing, Resuscitation Council (UK) (2007). *Decisions relating to cardiopulmonary resuscitation*. British Medical Association, London. https://www.resus.org.uk/dnacpr/decisions-relating-to-cpr (accessed 10 December 2019).

33. General Medical Council, *Treatment and care towards the end of life*.

34. NHS Scotland (2010). Do not attempt cardiopulmonary resuscitation (DNACPR): integrated adult policy: decision making and communication. https://www2.gov.scot/Publications/2010/05/24095633/1 (accessed 4 December 2019).

35. NHS Scotland (2016). Decisions about cardiopulmonary resuscitation: integrated adult policy. https://www.gov.scot/publications/decisions-cardiopulmonary-resuscitation-integrated-adult-policy (accessed 4 December 2019).

36. NHS Wales (2016). *A Clinical Policy for do Not Attempt Cardio Pulmonary Resuscitation (DNACPR) for Adults in Wales*. http://www.wales.nhs.uk/sitesplus/documents/862/134%20-DNACPR%20Policy%20English.pdf (accessed 4 December 2019).

37. National Confidential Enquiry into Patient Outcomes and Death (2012). *Time to intervene? A review of patients who underwent cardiopulmonary resuscitation as a result of in-hospital cardiorespiratory arrest*, at page 5. https://www.ncepod.org.uk/2012report1/downloads/CAP_fullreport.pdf (accessed 4 December 2019).

38. BMA, Resuscitation Council (UK), RCN, *Decisions relating to cardiopulmonary resuscitation*.

39. Ibid.

40. *Tracey*, at para 82.

41. NHS England (2017). *When seeing a specialist: your checklist*. https://www.nhs.uk/NHSEngland/AboutNHSservices/doctors/Documents/Print-ready_PatientReferral_PRINT.pdf (accessed 4 December 2019).

42. *Tracey*, at para 66.

43. House of Commons Health Committee (2015). Fifth Report of Session 2014–15, *End of Life Care*, HC 805, March, at para 58.

44. *Tracey*, at para 74.

45. *Tracey*, at para 86.

46. Callus T. (2017). One day I will find the right words, and they will be simple. *Journal of Public Health*, 1–5.

47. Fritz Z, Slowther A-M, Perkins GD. (2017). Resuscitation policy should focus on the patient, not the decision. *BMJ*, **356**, 1–8.

48. Perkins GD, Griffiths F, Slowther A-M, George R, Fritz Z, Satherley P, Williams B, Waugh N, Cooke MW, Chambers S, Mockford C, Freeman K, Grove A, Field R, Owen S, Clarke B, Court R, Hawkes C. (2016). Do-not-attempt-cardiopulmonary-resuscitation decisions: an evidence synthesis, *Health Services and Delivery Research*, **4(11)**. https://www.ncbi.nlm.nih.gov/books/NBK355498 (accessed 4 December 2019).

49. Fritz Z, Fuld J, Haydock S, Palmer C. (2010). Interpretation and intent: a study of the (mis)understanding of DNAR orders in a teaching hospital. *Resuscitation*, **81(9)**, 1138–41.

50. Clements M, Fuld J, Fritz Z. (2014). Documentation of resuscitation decision-making: a survey of practice in the United Kingdom. *Resuscitation*, **85**, 606–11.

51. Moffat S, Skinner J, Fritz Z. (2016). Does resuscitation status affect decision making in a deteriorating patient? Results from a randomised vignette study. *Journal of Evaluation in Clinical Practice*, **22(6)**, 917–23.

52. Henneman EA, Baird B, Bellamy PE, Rai G. (1994). Effect of do-not-resuscitate orders on the nursing care of critically ill patients. *American Journal of Critical Care*, **3**, 467–72.

53. Beach MC, Morrison RS. (2002). The effect of do-not-resuscitate orders on physician decision-making. *Journal of American Geriatric Soc*, **50**, 2057–61.

54. Mentzelopoulos S, Bossaert L, Raffay V, Askitopoulou H, Perkins GD, Grief R, Haywood K, Van de Voorde P. (2016). A survey of key opinion leaders on ethical resuscitation practices in 31 European countries. *Resuscitation*, **100**, 11–17.

55. O'Brien H, Scarlett S, Brady A, Harkin K, Kenny RA, Moriarty J. (2018). Do-not-attempt-resuscitation (DNAR) orders: understanding and interpretation of their use in the hospitalised patient in Ireland. A brief report. Journal of Medical Ethics, **44**, 201–3, at 201.

56. Ibid, at 203.

57. Kazaure H, Roman S, Sosa JA. (2011). High mortality in surgical patients with do-not-resuscitate orders: analysis of 8256 patients. *Archives of Surgery*, **146**, 922–8.

58. Cohn S, Fritz ZBM, Frankau JM, Laroche CM, Fuld JP. (2013). Do not attempt cardiopulmonary resuscitation (DNACPR) orders in acute medical settings: a qualitative study. *QJM*, **106(2)**, 165–77.

59. Baskett PJ, Lim A. (2004). The varying ethical attitudes towards resuscitation in Europe. Resuscitation, **62**, 267–73.

60. Mentzelopoulos et al., A survey of key opinion leaders.

61. Baskett PJ, et al. The varying ethical attitudes.

62. Mentzelopoulos et al., A survey of key opinion leaders.

63. Council of Europe (2015). *Guide on the decision-making process regarding medical treatment in end-of-life situations.* https://www.coe.int/en/web/bioethics/guide-on-the-decision-making-process-regarding-medical-treatment-in-end-of-life-situations (accessed 4 December 2019).

64. Oviedo Convention, ETS No. 164, 1997.

65. Council of Europe, *Guide on the decision-making process*, at page 9.

66. Fritz Z, Fuld J. (2015). Development of the Universal Form of Treatment Options (UFTO) as an alternative to Do Not Attempt Cardiopulmonary Resuscitation (DNACPR) orders: a cross-disciplinary approach. *Journal of Education in Clinical Practice*, **21(1)**, 109–17.

67. Fritz et al., Interpretation and intent.

68. Cohn et al., Do not attempt cardiopulmonary resuscitation orders in acute medical settings.
69. Department of Health (2014). *Older people – service framework documents.* https://www.health-ni.gov.uk/publications/older-people-service-framework-documents (accessed 4 December 2019).
70. *Re T (Adult) (Refusal of Medical Treatment)* [1992] 4 All ER 649.
71. *Re MB* [1997] 2 FLR 426.
72. https://www.resus.org.uk/respect (accessed 21 December 2019).
73. Oliver D. (2017). Why I'm changing my mind about resuscitation. *BMJ*, **356**, j1143. https://doi.org/10.1136/bmj.j1143 (accessed 4 December 2019).
74. *Tracey*, at para 92.
75. Fritz Z, Cork N, Dodd A, et al. (2014). DNACPR decisions: challenging and changing practice in the wake of the Tracey judgment, *Clinical Medicine*, **14**, 571–6.
76. *McFarlane v Tayside Health Board* [2000] 2 AC 59 HL.
77. BMA, RCN, Resuscitation Council (UK), *Decisions relating to cardiopulmonary resuscitation*, at page 10.
78. *Ms B v An NHS Trust* [2002] EWHC 429.
79. Michalowski S. (2007). Trial and error at the end of life: no harm done? *Oxford Journal of Legal Studies*, **27**(2), 257–80.
80. Paduano M. (2017). Payout after woman was kept alive against her will, BBC News, 6 December https://www.bbc.co.uk/news/uk-england-coventry-warwickshire-42240148 (accessed 4 December 2019).
81. *Re T (Adult: Refusal of Treatment)* [1993] Fam 95 CA at 117.
82. *Malette v Shulman* (1990) 67 DLR (4th) 321.
83. *Anderson v St Francis-St George Hospital, inc.*, 671NE 2d 225 (Ohio 1996).
84. *Allore v Flower Hospital* 699 NE 2d 560 (Ohio App6th Dist. 1997).
85. Michalowski, Trial and error at the end of life.
86. Strasser M. (1999). A jurisprudence in disarray: on battery, wrongful living and the right to bodily integrity. *San Diego Law Review*, 997–1041.
87. Knapp W, Hamilton F. (1992). 'Wrongful living': resuscitation as tortuous interference with a patient's right to give informed refusal. *Northern Kentucky Law Review*, **19**(2), 253–77.
88. *Chester v Afshar* [2004] UKHL 41.
89. *R (Burke) v General Medical Council* [2005] EWCA Civ 1003.
90. *Re J (A Minor) (Wardship: Medical Treatment)* [1990] 3 All 930.
91. BMA, RCN, Resuscitation Council (UK), *Decisions relating to cardiopulmonary resuscitation*.
92. Campbell R. (2017). Do not attempt cardiopulmonary resuscitation decisions: joint guidance. *J R Coll Physicians*, **47**, 47–51, at 48.

93. Price D. (2009). What shape euthanasia after Bland? Historical, contemporary and futuristic paradigms. *Law Quarterly Review*, **125**(1), 142–74, at 152.

94. Wilson J. (2008). To what extent should older patients be included in decisions regarding their resuscitation status? *Journal of Medical Ethics*, **34**, 353–6.

95. Morgan D. (1994). Odysseus and the binding directive: only a cautionary tale. *Legal Studies*, **14**(3), 411–42.

96. *Re R (Adult: Medical Treatment)* [1996] 2 FLR 99.

97. *R (Burke) v General Medical Council* [2005] EWCA Civ 1003.

98. Ibid.

99. *Re J (A, Minor) (Wardship: Medical Treatment)* [1993] 3 All ER 930.

100. *University Hospitals Birmingham Foundation Trust v HB and FB* [2018] EWCOP 39.

101. For example, Hull L. (2008). Family's fury as they discover 'do not resuscitate' order in mother's file after she dies. *The Daily Mail*, 25 March. http://www.dailymail.co.uk/news/article-543374/Family's-fury-discover-resuscitate-order-mothers-file-dies.html (accessed 4 December 2019).

102. Hill ME, MacQuillan G, Forsyth M, Heath DA. (1994). Cardiopulmonary resuscitation: who makes the decision? *BMJ*, **308**, 1677.

103. Morgan R, King D, Prajapati C, Rowe J. (1994). Views of elderly patients and their relatives on cardiopulmonary resuscitation. *BMJ*, **308**, 1677–8.

104. Manisty C, Waxman J. (2003). Doctors should not discuss resuscitation with terminally ill patients. *BMJ*, **327**, 614–15.

105. Fritz et al., Development of the Universal Form of Treatment Options.

PART B

LISTENING TO DOCTORS, PARENTS, AND RELATIVES

4

Spanner in the Works or Cogs in a Wheel?

Parents and Decision Making for Critically Ill Young Children

Thérèse Callus

Introduction

Paediatric intensive care units all around the world bear witness to complex decisions regarding the withdrawing or withholding of life-sustaining treatment for children.[1] The decision is never going to be an easy one, but a professional and legal framework of shared and collaborative decision making based around the deceptively attractive notion of the child's 'best interests' means that, for the most part, such difficult decisions are usually agreed by all the parties involved. Despite the indeterminate nature of best interests and, as we shall see below, the intersection of statutory guidance and common law, there is support[2] for the notion of best interests to provide a flexible and case-specific response that recognizes that 'every case and every child is unique'.[3] Therefore, even when conflicts may arise between treating clinicians and parents, the vast majority of them will be resolved without requiring the intervention of a court.[4]

Nevertheless, with technological advances permitting life to be prolonged even with the bleakest of prognosis, the sensitive and challenging question of limiting treatment has become more acute. The latest framework from the Royal College of Paediatrics and Child Health identifies three main categories of situation in which treatment of a critically ill child may be limited: (1) where life is limited in quantity; (2) where life is limited in quality; and (3) where a child may be deemed competent to refuse proposed treatment and prefer palliative care.[5] All decisions are founded on 'shared knowledge and mutual respect' but are universally recognized as involving a complex web of medical, emotional, social, and familial issues. Inevitably, conflict may arise but the overarching aim is to find as much common ground as possible. Rarely, such common ground may become negligible and, if so, the conflict escalates beyond the confines of the doctor–patient relationship.

From time to time, mass media attention focuses on a small number of such intractable disputes between parents of critically ill young children and the treating medical team.[6] All too often, increasingly emotive and polarized stands ensue, and the complex issues at play become confused and concealed. But it is not only the general public who struggle with this situation. Medical practitioners, ethicists, and lawyers do not all agree on the optimal course of action, or indeed on the principles that should guide any decision making in these cases.[7] In this chapter, I set out the legal and professional frameworks for such decision making, highlighting areas of broad consensus and engaging with the more controversial and differing opinions on the appropriateness of the current position. While I concentrate on the treatment of babies and young children—who by definition are unable to participate in the decision-making process—I also include, where relevant, considerations relative to older children, so-called 'mature minors'.

I start with the principle that, in general, parents will make decisions for their critically ill young children with advice and support from the treating medical team. After all, parents have a duty to care for their children. However, for older children, both the Mental Capacity Act 2005, which applies to incompetent 16–17-year-olds, and a court's inherent jurisdiction, which can be invoked up to 18 years of age, come into play. Compatibility between the statute and the common law for this latter group remains problematic, as does the status of the parent as a decision maker.[8]

The second part examines when the parties cannot agree and make an application to the High Court to resolve the conflict. I then discuss how the court adopts the concept of best interests to arrive at a decision, which is very much fact-dependent and open to different interpretations. Given that we acknowledge parents are usually best placed to make decisions concerning their child, it is not axiomatic that—just because their decision might not align with that of the medical team—it should be questioned. Some argue for the best interests test to be replaced with a 'significant harm' test, but this appears to merely replace one nebulous concept with another. In order to alleviate the perception that it is a binary decision between an unacceptable and a best outcome, in the final section I suggest framing the question in terms of 'not against the child's interest', or, indeed, what is 'compatible' with the child's interests.[9]

Parents as primary decision makers?

> [W]hile there is now no rule of law that the rights and wishes of unimpeachable parents must prevail over other considerations, such rights and wishes, recognised as they are by nature and society, can be capable of ministering to the total welfare of the child in a special way, and must therefore preponderate in many cases. The parental rights, however, remain qualified and not absolute ... [10]

In what circumstances should medical treatment decisions concerning a child be treated differently from any one of a myriad of important decisions that parents routinely make for their children without any state intervention?

Young children

It is perhaps trite to say that, in general, parents, or at least those with parental responsibility,[11] will make the decision relating to their child's treatment that is generally understood to be in the child's best interests. After all, they are expected to be the best placed to do this, given their intimate knowledge of the child, their shared life together, and their (usually) loving bond. Their decision will be informed and supported by the treating clinical team. This emphasis on shared decision making is well entrenched in medical practice, and professional guidelines underline the need for the clinical team to pay due respect to parents' beliefs and values.[12] One example of this can be seen in the case of *Tafida Raqeeb v Barts NHS Foundation Trust* where MacDonald J held that:

> the court should give weight to the reflection that in the last analysis the best interests of every child include an expectation that difficult decisions affecting the length and quality of the child's life will be taken for the child by a parent in the exercise of their parental responsibility.[13]

In this case, the question of whether it was in the child's best interests to continue to be ventilated included consideration of the parents' deeply held religious views, which, it was suggested, would be likely to be shared by the child (at least as far as the child's level of maturity would allow). Such thinking recognizes the private nature of such decisions, which should, unless there is good reason not to, remain immune from external intervention from the state. Indeed, as Baker J stated in the case of Ashya King:

> ... the State – whether it be the court, or any other public authority – has no business interfering with the exercise of parental responsibility unless the child is suffering or is likely to suffer significant harm as a result of the care given to the child not being what it would be reasonable to expect a parent to give.[14]

In this case, the hospital trust offered the established treatment for the boy's condition. However, the parents sought an alternative, which they believed offered the optimal outcome for their child with the least potential side effects, but which was not available in the UK. Fearful that the trust would prevent them from taking their child abroad for treatment, the parents removed the him from the hospital without the doctors' knowledge. A much publicized search followed and ultimately an arrest warrant for the parents was effected in Spain. The child was made a ward of court. It transpired through the course of the hearing that the parents felt that all communication channels between themselves and the treating hospital in the UK had broken down, and that the hospital would thwart their attempts to provide the innovative treatment for their son abroad, given that it was not available in the UK on the NHS at that time. It is evident that the intention of the parents was merely to enable the provision of a type of treatment, for which they had secured funding, and also that it was a treatment option that, according to the judge, was viable. Because the court recognized the viability of the treatment the parents sought, and their right to choose, there was no comparative analysis of which treatment would be in the child's best interests.

In effect, this reflects what happens on a daily basis for most decisions concerning children, where, unless a parent's action is said to go against the interests of the child, the state does not dictate that one option is preferable to another. We see this in decisions as varied as the selection of a school, the choice of religion, or the decision whether to vaccinate a child.[15] However, we cannot ignore the fact that, occasionally, a parent's decision may actually harm a child[16] and that, where a child is suffering or likely to suffer significant harm, the state will intervene.[17] Despite respect for personal values and beliefs, trust in divine healing, for example, will no longer exonerate a parent from not allowing the necessary medical treatment. So, although in the nineteenth century, parents who relied on divine intervention at the expense of treating their child were found not guilty of manslaughter,[18] later cases show that parents will be pursued through the criminal law (and, where proven, found guilty) when they have put their child's life in danger by rejecting the necessary medical treatment.[19] Some argue, therefore, that, unless it can be shown that the child is suffering or likely to suffer significant harm as a result of the parents' decision, the parents should hold the decision-making power. I examine later the difference between these two approaches and their potential overlap. But first we should also note that the dispute can sometimes be between the parents themselves. Doctors may propose treatment that one parent agrees with but the other does not. Likewise, a parent may request feasible treatment but the other parent may object. In both cases, the legal position of the doctor is relatively clear: where they have the consent of one parent, then they are permitted to proceed provided they believe the treatment to be in the child's interests.[20] Indeed, 'If the parents disagree, one consenting and the other refusing, the doctor will be presented with a professional and ethical, but not with a legal problem because if he has the consent of one authorized person, treatment will not without more constitute a trespass or a criminal assault'.[21] However, it is recognized that, when treatment decisions have serious and potentially lifelong consequences, no doctor would proceed without authorization from a court.[22]

Adolescents and 16–18-year-olds

The role of parents in decision making for older children—who may have a view on the treatment that is being proposed, and an ability to express themselves—requires further examination. The Family Law Reform Act 1969 provides that those aged 16 and over can give valid consent to surgical, mental, or dental treatment, and that in such cases parental consent is not needed.[23] Furthermore, the Mental Capacity Act 2005 applies the same presumption of capacity to 16- and 17-year-olds as for adults. Whether parents can override a refusal by a competent 16- or 17-year-old has been described by Baroness Hale as a 'controversial' question.[24] However, it remains the case that a court may override a competent minor's refusal, under its inherent jurisdiction, declaring that life-sustaining treatment is lawful. Such was the outcome in *Re P*[25] where the court found itself under a duty to declare lawful treatment that would prevent the death of a competent but gravely ill 17-year-old, citing primarily its duty under article 2 European Convention on Human Rights (ECHR) to preserve life.[26]

Following the decision of the Supreme Court in *Re D (A Child)*, it is now clear that parents cannot seek to bring about the confinement of their 16- or 17-year-old child for purposes of receiving treatment.[27] In that case, the majority of the Supreme Court held that, when a young adult of 16- or

17-years-old is not able to consent to being confined (that is, being subject to continuous supervision and control, and not being free to leave a particular place), that 16- or 17-year-old should be seen to be deprived of liberty for purposes of Article 5 ECHR. The Supreme Court made clear that this would be the case even if the child's parents sought to authorize the position by giving their consent. The logic of that decision would apply equally—indeed even more strongly—to the position where the child *has* the capacity to make a decision whether to consent or refuse the confinement and refuses to consent. The Supreme Court expressly declined to address issues wider than confinement, but it is likely that the courts will be asked to reflect sooner rather than later whether consideration of treatment in relation to 16–17-year-olds with impaired decision-making capacity should be undertaken by reference to s4 Mental Capacity Act 2005, rather than by reference to whether the parents are consenting (or refusing) treatment on behalf of their child.

With respect to children under 16-years-old, the case of *Gillick* recognized that they can consent to treatment that is offered by a doctor (and therefore presumed to be in their best interests) provided that they are found to be competent for the purposes of the decision being taken[28]—in effect, that they understand the nature of the proposed treatment and its likely consequences. The parental duty therefore 'dwindles'. For 'Gillick competent' minors, their refusal can be overridden, not by the parents but by the court's interpretation of the adolescent's best interests under the exercise of its inherent jurisdiction, and this irrespective of the parents' wishes.[29]

However, in all situations, there is some evolution in the appreciation of best interests on the basis that the courts are adopting a more subjective approach to interpreting best interests along the lines of that applied to adults, placing the assumed wishes and feelings of the patient (irrespective of age) at the heart of their decisions, and at the same time reducing the role of parents' views. There is evidence of this concerning both very young babies[30] and older children[31] but, as we shall see later, its suitability for children is questionable. Clearly, there are complex issues at stake in deciding upon important medical treatment and whether it concerns babies, young children, or older adolescents, in the case of a dispute, the court is at present the principal forum in which conflict is addressed. How then is the court involved?

Making an application to the court

It follows from the previous section that when the parents (and, when competent, the child) and the medical team are in agreement, then there will be no need to seek the intervention of a court.[32] This is in contrast to the previous situation concerning adults, when it was believed that if the action involved withholding or withdrawing life-sustaining treatment, such as artificial hydration and nutrition, then a declaration as to the lawfulness of such withdrawal should be sought from a court.[33] However, the Supreme Court in *Re Y* has confirmed that, just as for children, when there is no conflict between the treating team and the patient's family, there is no need to seek a declaration from a court as to the lawfulness of the proposed withdrawal of treatment.[34] However, in the face of an intractable dispute that cannot be resolved within the treating team, or subsequently within a wider hospital multi-disciplinary team or mediation, then an application should be made to a court to resolve the issue:

> There has been some public concern as to why the court is involved at all. We do not ask for work but we have a duty to decide what parties with a proper interest ask us to decide. […] The only arbiter of that sincerely held difference of opinion is the court. Deciding disputed matters of life and death is surely and pre-eminently a matter for a court of law to judge. That is what courts are here for.[35]

Both the General Medical Council guidelines[36] and the case law[37] confirm this. Notably, the case of *Glass v UK* before the European Court of Human Rights underlined the requirement—in the case of dispute—for the hospital trust to make an application to the High Court as to the legality of the proposed treatment. Although the message is clear as to the need to involve the court, and the onus being on the hospital trust to make the application, there nevertheless remain questions as to when an application should be made, whether it should be to invoke the inherent jurisdiction of the court, or an application for an explicit child arrangements order under the Children Act 1989.[38] In the case of Alfie Evans, the court held that an approach that combines both a s8 specific issue order and declaratory relief under the inherent jurisdiction is preferable.[39]

Given the often critical condition of the children, the timing of an application can be problematic. In *Re OT*,[40] a 10-month-old boy suffered from a serious mitochondrial condition that left him dependent on a ventilator, having suffered a stroke, and with brain stem damage. Doctors sought a declaration that it would be lawful to remove the boy from ventilation and to administer palliative care. The parents sought an adjournment to seek other expert opinion, but this was refused. On appeal, the court found that the hospital had not delayed unduly in making its application, noting that there was a balance to be found between '(a) applying in advance of a crisis when the exact medical evidence may be subject to some revision; and (b) waiting for a time which is nearer the crisis but with all the practical problems of a rushed hearing.'[41]

Timing was also central in the case of Charlie Gard. Charlie, although born apparently healthy, was admitted to hospital at 8 weeks old and was never discharged. He was diagnosed with a very rare inherited mitochondrial depletion syndrome, a progressive and fatal disease affecting his ability to both physically and mentally function. There is no cure for the disease, but the parents had researched the possibility of him undergoing experimental nucleoside therapy, which had only been tried for a different mitochondrial condition. His treating team had prepared a request to the rapid response clinical ethics committee for this therapy but, before a decision was taken, Charlie suffered what clinicians agreed was serious, irreversible brain damage. Consequently, the treating team, weighing up the advantages and disadvantages of maintaining Charlie on a ventilator in order to access the therapy that was not of certain benefit, decided that this would not be in his best interests. A second medical opinion confirmed this. Faced with a contrary position from Charlie's parents, who felt Charlie should have 'one last shot', the hospital sought a declaration from the court that it was not in Charlie's best interests to undergo the nucleoside therapy (which had been offered by a doctor in the US), and that it would be legal for ventilation to be withdrawn and palliative care provided. Because of the adversarial nature of the litigation and the appeals by the parents against the declarations made by the lower courts, a not insignificant period of time lapsed, during which time Charlie's condition deteriorated. Each stage thereby required a stay of the initial declaration and the doctors continued to treat Charlie, even though they did not believe it was in his best interests. The delay was increased by an application to the European Court of Human Rights, which found the parents' case inadmissible.[42]

The question that follows is whether a court is the best placed to make a decision in the face of conflict between parents and clinicians. In some circumstances, the length and nature of litigation mean that the outcome satisfies no-one—the process is emotionally draining for both the parents and the treating team, and delay can both force a doctor to continue treating against clinical judgment and prolong the ultimate outcome of a decision by which the parents will lose their child. On the other hand, one advantage could be said to be the wider implication of a court decision. Inherent in each judgment is a public statement of potential interest to all, and one which may, depending on the level of the court, provide a precedent or at least a guide for future decision-making situations. As expressed by Hedley J in the Charlotte Wyatt case:

> Any civilised society must have the means by which intractable disputes, whether
> between the State and the citizen, or between citizens themselves, are to be re-
> solved. That is the purpose of the Courts and the system of civil and family justice
> in this country. […] It may well be that an external decision is in the end a better
> solution than the stark alternatives of medical or parental veto.[43]

Nevertheless, general agreement on a court being involved does not hide the
very real difficulties associated with making a decision concerning the appropriate treatment for a patient. It is acknowledged that a patient (or their family)
cannot insist on treatment that a doctor believes is not in their best interests.[44]
Likewise, a court will not order a doctor to continue or refrain from treating
when the doctor believes that the treatment is futile.[45] But, in such a case, a patient should be referred to a doctor who would be willing to offer or withdraw
the treatment if the court believes that it would be in the patient's best interests
to do so.[46] In making decisions as to the lawfulness of treatment, the court refers to the overarching objective of whether it is in the patient's best interests
to give the treatment. As Baroness Hale stated in *Aintree*:

> the focus is on whether it is in the patient's best interests to give the treatment,
> rather than on whether it is in his best interests to withhold or withdraw it. If the
> treatment is not in his best interests, the court will not be able to give its consent on
> his behalf and it will follow that it will be lawful to withhold or withdraw it. Indeed,
> it will follow that it will not be lawful to give it.[47]

While relating to an adult patient lacking capacity, this has been explicitly
applied in cases concerning children.[48] Yet, while intuitively attractive, the
best interests concept is far from easy to assess, as the sometimes apparently
contradictory judicial explanations reveal.

Best interests—a legal concept

As noted in the introduction, there is no statutory definition of best interests
per se, but there are statutory guidelines that indicate a range of factors that
may be relevant to making a best interests decision. Both s4 Mental Capacity
Act 2005 (for incapacitated adults and 16–17-year-olds) and s1(3) Children
Act 1989 (when the court exercises its inherent jurisdiction or grants an order
under s8 of the Act for anyone up to age 18) contain such a list. However, it
is important to note that, whereas the Mental Capacity Act deals specifically

with medical decision making, the Children Act's application is far more general and the s1(3) checklist does not particularly lend itself to the context of serious medical treatment decisions. Notably, in cases concerning treatment for children, the court does not tend to explicitly invoke the checklist under s1(3).

In the context of treatment for incapacitated adults, Baroness Hale held that in establishing best interests,

> [T]he most that can be said, therefore, is that [...] decision-makers must look at his welfare in the widest sense, not just medical but social and psychological; they must consider the nature of the medical treatment in question, what it involves and its prospects of success; they must consider what the outcome of that treatment for the patient is likely to be; they must try and put themselves in the place of the individual patient and ask what his attitude to the treatment is or would be likely to be; and they must consult others who are looking after him or interested in his welfare, in particular for their view of what his attitude would be.[49]

This has been applied in the same way to considering the best interests of children, although the extent to which a child's attitude can be discerned is debatable.[50] In *Re MB*, the court insisted that there is an objective approach to best interests, which must be judged from the child's perspective. The court does not 'step into the shoes of the parent',[51] or decide what they would do if in the child's position,[52] although asking what the child's views are, or would be, is not so far removed from the latter. Thus, there is some controversy as to whether it is (or ever could be) an objective assessment. Inevitably, we have to acknowledge that there is a subjective element that has been strongly supported by the Supreme Court in the context of treatment for incapacitated adults, as illustrated in the David James case and reiterated in the case of Tafida Raqeeb where it was held: ' ... where a child is not in pain and is not aware of his or her parlous situation, these cases can place the objective best interests test under some stress. Absent the fact of pain or the awareness of suffering, the answer to the objective best interests tests must be looked for in subjective or highly value laden ethical, moral or religious factors extrinsic to the child, such as futility (in its nontechnical sense), dignity, the meaning of life and the principle of the sanctity of life, which factors mean different things to different people in a diverse, multicultural, multifaith society'.[53] The starting point in cases concerning treatment for a child is the 'assumed point of view of the patient'[54] and we have cases where the court asks itself what the child *would* want. In the case of a severely injured two-year-old who was dependent upon ventilation with little prospect of improvement, the Court of

Appeal confirmed that the first instance judge's assertion that: 'I do not think that A would want this life for himself' was a relevant consideration.[55] In the same vein, but with the contrary conclusion, MacDonald J in *Tafida Raqeeb v Barts NHS Foundation Trust* stated that he was 'satisfied that if Tafida was asked she would not reject out of hand a situation in which she continued to live, albeit in a moribund and at best minimally conscious state, without pain and in the loving care of her dedicated family, consistent with her formative appreciation that life is precious, a wish to follow a parent's religious practice and a non-judgmental attitude to disability'.[56] Indeed, we should be mindful that 'even very severely handicapped people find a quality of life rewarding which to the unhandicapped may seem manifestly intolerable. People have an amazing adaptability'.[57] So, despite the 'easily stated and universally applauded'[58] notion of best interests, the exercise is more complex than it first appears. What is clear is that the test goes beyond best clinical interests to include 'medical, emotional and all other welfare issues' of the child,[59] and tends to now include greater emphasis on their purported wishes and feelings. This trend has been underscored by commentary on the Convention on the Rights of Persons with Disabilities insofar as the best interests test is perceived as failing to accord sufficient weight to the wishes and values of a person lacking capacity.[60]

There is clearly a balancing exercise to be carried out, one in which ' ... a surrogate decision maker must determine the highest net benefit among the available options, assigning different weights to interests the patient has in each option and discounting or subtracting inherent risks or costs'.[61] This approach, based upon a 'balance sheet' of advantages and disadvantages of the proposed treatment or withdrawal of treatment, is one that the English judges have adopted, albeit with a level of caution indicating that a balance sheet simpliciter may not adequately convey the respective weight of individual factors. It should be seen as an 'aide memoire', not a substitute for reasoned judgment.[62] In some cases, such an exercise may be relatively straightforward. For example, when a blood transfusion would save a child's life but the parents object on the grounds of their religious faith as Jehovah Witnesses, a court will tend to declare that such treatment is in the child's best interests and therefore lawful.[63] Likewise, even when faced with a *Gillick* competent minor, a court will usually apply best interests as requiring life to be preserved and will overrule the child's refusal.[64] For an incompetent 16- or 17-year-old, the court could declare treatment lawful as in the adolescent's best interests under s4 Mental Capacity Act 2005, although the focus on what the court believes the child's wishes would have been will be more prominent and could potentially result in the decision not to declare the treatment lawful if the court establishes that the child, if competent, would not have wanted to go ahead with it. Despite the superficial attraction of the balance sheet, it may conceal unconscious value opinions and not translate the purported views of the patient themselves. Although there is a presumption in favour of action that will prolong life, the courts have accepted that 'to prolong life is not the sole objective of the court and to require it at the expense of other considerations may not be in the child's best interest'.[65] But there is the risk that the court simply substitutes its judgment over that of the parent, or indeed what the child might have wanted. There is also a wider familial perspective that is inextricably bound up with the child.[66] In *Re MB*, Holman J refused to declare that it would be lawful to withdraw ventilation, citing the important bond between the child and his family from which the child may have felt some benefit.[67]

Unilateral decision making ultimately by a judge is open to further criticism on the basis that it lacks moral authority, especially if it is difficult to ascertain what the patient's own view would be. Why is the judge's interpretation of what the child would want any more valid than that of their parents or the doctors?[68] Some academic arguments appear to favour at least a presumption that, when there is a choice of possible options, the parents' choice should be respected. Ranaan Gillon forcefully argued that for Charlie Gard. There were two morally defensible outcomes: either the judge could rule as he did, that an assessment of the child's best interests meant that it would be lawful for ventilation to be withdrawn; or, alternatively, that it would be lawful for the current medical team to hand over Charlie's care and treatment to another team that was willing to try the experimental treatment for Charlie.[69] For Gillon, there could not be said to be an objective assessment of best interests. Nevertheless, this argument is weakened by the factual reality that, in the Gard case, experimental treatment was very unlikely to offer any benefit to Charlie at all. Furthermore, protracted litigation to establish what is in a child's best interests paradoxically may go against all sides' respective interpretations of how best to protect the welfare of the child. As Baroness Hale remarked in the Gard case, the delays made the judiciary 'complicit in directing a course of action which is contrary to Charlie's best interests'.[70]

Despite a wider interpretation of best interests to encompass emotional, social, and familial aspects of a child's welfare, the weight of medical evidence in critical care cases cannot be ignored. Yet, when faced with competing interpretations of a child's best interests by those who all claim to know what is best, when should the parental decision not be decisive? Further, how appropriate can it be to transpose the focus on the wishes and feelings of an incapacitated adult within the context of young children who may never have had the opportunity to comprehend, much less express themselves on, their condition?

How can the judge's (or anyone else's) interpretation of what the child would want be justified? Should we accord primacy to the clinical recommendation? Faced with these difficulties, some suggest that the notion of 'harm' could be an alternative mechanism that would better balance both the interests of critically ill children and those of the parents in remaining, at least presumptively, the ones best placed to take decisions relating to their child's treatment.[71] The Ashya King case seems to open up this direction. But is it a better option?

Reframing best interests?

Perhaps the greatest harm to critically ill children is to allow disputes concerning their treatment to be aired in the court of public opinion. Issues become clouded and tensions increase. One argument put forward to support parents' position that they should be free to decide if their child receives treatment elsewhere is based upon the notion that, unless the child is suffering, or at risk of suffering significant harm, parents should remain the primary decision makers. This equates with the significant harm threshold test applied to justify state intervention in a child's upbringing.[72] So the question is not what is the best outcome for the child but rather what is necessary to avoid the child from suffering from harm. The state—be it the court or the treating hospital—should not interfere with the parents' desire to take their child elsewhere for treatment unless it is shown that the child would suffer significant harm as a result. Charlie Gard's parents argued that he was not at risk of significant harm by the proposed move to access experimental treatment in the US. They claimed there was a slight chance that it could at least restrict his decline and was a viable course of treatment. But it was found at first instance, and reiterated by the Court of Appeal, that 'such treatment would be futile, by which I mean would be of no effect *but may well cause pain, suffering and distress to* Charlie' (emphasis added).[73] Reliance upon the Ashya King case, as suggested by counsel for the parents, was misplaced insofar as there was no real conflict as to the choice of treatment in Charlie's case.[74] So, even if we apply the harm threshold, we would have nevertheless come to the same outcome as the best interest test. The argument was further elaborated for Alfie Evans whereby counsel for the parents submitted that, to justify the court's intervention in the decision-making process, it must be shown that the child would suffer significant harm from the parents' own decision. They claimed that they were treated unfairly when the court exercised its inherent jurisdiction, compared to parents whom the State considers are not suitable to care for their own children in proceedings under s31 Children Act 1989.[75] However, the court rejected this comparison, preferring to equate the position of parents under the inherent jurisdiction with that under s8 proceedings, whereby both are subject to the best interests principle.[76] This must surely be the correct comparator insofar as the purpose behind the s31 Children Act threshold is to justify state intervention when parents are found to be acting contrary to their child's interests. In the context of medical treatment or withdrawal, the purpose of intervention must be to decide on the optimal treatment for the child when faced with conflicting views between parents and doctors.

Empirical studies on harm confirm that it is not a better mechanism for addressing conflict in treatment decisions. Giles Birchley's systematic review of the harm threshold in treatment decisions for children, when the parents and treating team are in disagreement, identified that a test of harm suffers from the same indeterminacy as best interests.[77] Moreover, he alludes to the evaluative nature of the term 'harm'. Indeed, I would suggest that the term 'harm' may itself be harmful insofar as it tends to suggest that there is an element of condemnable fault. If a court has to evaluate whether the parents' decision would cause 'harm', a positive finding to this effect might suggest that the parents are in some way culpable. Such an approach clearly has no place in the sensitive question of the appropriate treatment of a critically ill child. Best interests—imperfect as it may be—does nevertheless remove any suggestion of fault or substandard care on behalf of the parents, and talks to the ideal of finding the best solution in a bleak situation. Furthermore, the notion of harm is not absent from the best interests assessment. Indeed, under the welfare checklist in s1(3) Children Act 1989, the court is directed to consider any harm the child is suffering, or is likely to suffer. Consequently, harm, just like intolerability, may be invoked as one of several elements to elucidate whether treatment would best further the child's interests, without elevating it to a threshold criterion.

Yet one difficulty with the notion of 'best interests' is that it implies that there is only one 'right' answer. Reference to the Children Act's 'welfare' checklist leaves scope to develop our thinking on best interests and suggest that an alternative 'not against the child's interests' test could prove to be a more accessible and acceptable approach to decision making for sick children. By asking whether the treatment proposed or refused by the parents would go against the child's interests would negate the need to identify only one acceptable outcome. Moreover, it would place more emphasis on the *process* of decision making, which is arguably as important as the test itself, as Jo Bridgman has also identified.[78] By reframing the question in terms of which options are feasible because they do not go against the child's interests, we might encourage greater use of mediation and encourage an environment where the outcome is not simply binary—between the 'best' and 'unacceptable' outcomes. Given parents' ability to research alternative options that may be available elsewhere, a forum where these could be explored together could be helpful. By way of comparison, the procedural-focused French system suggests that automatic use of hospital ethics committees is one of the main reasons behind the lack of litigation in this area in France. There, a case involving the withdrawal of life-sustaining treatment on an 18-month-old child highlights the centrality of process over potential conflict about interests. In the case of *Marwa*, although the Conseil d'Etat (the supreme administrative court) did not declare lawful the withdrawal of artificial nutrition and hydration for the child, as requested by the medical team, the justification for the decision lay not in preferring the parents' interpretation of the child's interest in being kept alive but rather the need to allow a reasonable delay before withdrawal of Clinically Assisted Nutrition and Hydration in order to explore all the options.[79] Despite some reform in France concerning end of life treatment that suggests greater weight is being given to the patient's own views (or those of a child's parents), the law nevertheless focuses on the collegial procedure within the medical corps to ensure that any treatment decision can be justified.[80] Consequently, there appears to be a notable dearth of reported cases of conflict between parents and medical teams. This can be explained by the fact that the process involved is necessarily multi-disciplinary and includes use of ethics committees and mediation. Further, the strict procedural guidelines include the need for a period of time to elapse between bleak prognosis and the actual withdrawal of treatment. This time can be spent in helping parents and families to accept and understand the futility of continued treatment, with a focus on support and mediation.[81]

However, it is clear that no extra level of mediation or arbitration will be effective unless all the parties sign up to the possibility that the committee will ultimately find in favour of a solution that may not be what one party wanted, or believed to be in the child's interest. But there is support for the option of a strengthened ethical forum to encourage agreement. Huxtable refers to specialist ethics services that could prevent conflict and allow deeper engagement with the ethical element of decisions concerning life-sustaining treatment.[82] Hain has proposed a 'children's interests panel', which would include both medics and lawyers, and, he suggests, be legally binding.[83] Others have suggested that a lower tier of tribunal could address some of the difficulties inherent in litigation before the courts, while maintaining the advantages of independent adjudication.[84] Francis J at first instance in the Gard case noted:

> I believe that it would, in all cases like this, be helpful for there to be some form of issues resolution hearing or other form of mediation where the parties can have confidential conversations to see what common ground can be reached between

them. I believe that that type of hearing, be it judge-led or some other form of private mediation, would have led to a greater understanding between the parents and the clinical team in this case.[85]

At the UK's leading children's hospital, Great Ormond Street (GOSH) in London, a clinical ethics service (CES) has been developed since 2012, resulting in a dedicated ethics service commended by the Care Quality Commission in 2016.[86] However, any extra layer to aid discussion and agreement between parties requires resourcing. The CES at GOSH exists predominantly due to charitable funding and extended voluntary contributions by professionals. Furthermore, delays in the use of such a service, or the belief by parents that the service is not impartial, may negate its potential effectiveness (as happened in the case of Charlie Gard).

Trials using conflict management models in paediatric care have also been shown to be relatively effective in avoiding the 'conflict pathway'[87] between medical professionals and parents. In one trial, the conflict management model adopted was effective in reducing the incidence of conflict and was deemed to be acceptable to medical professionals.[88] The model is comprised of two phases: phase 1 helps to identify potential conflict triggers and allows a communication plan to be drawn up with the family to better manage expectations; phase 2 is invoked when communication has broken down, and includes involvement of senior hospital staff. However, even when there are conflict management models and alternative dispute resolution avenues, other issues may also be at play. All fora require relevant evidence and, as Bridgman has identified, timely production of feasible evidence as to viable alternative options is needed for resolution of disagreement. This is particularly difficult when it concerns experimental treatment. Indeed, with immediate and widespread access to information from around the world, the existence of experimental therapy poses a particular problem, as does the use of 'expert' opinions from multiple sources. As in many cases, the prospect of any chance or hope (however unrealistic or unfeasible in practice) is one that desperate parents will latch onto in the hope of some benefit for their child. At present, the law is clear that experimental therapy should only be considered when there can be shown some 'direct benefit' for the child themselves.[89] But note that guidance from the Royal College of Paediatrics states that parents can consent to research procedures 'if the risks are sufficiently small to mean that the research can be reasonably said not to go against the child's interests'.[90] Likewise, the Nuffield Council on Bioethics suggests that parents could consent to clinical research which is *compatible* with their child's immediate and longer-term welfare. Yet access to, and funding for, experimental treatment is complex—should parents who are able to pay for treatment be allowed to try anything in their search for improvement in their child's condition? What are the implications of such populist approaches to crowd funding, such as that generated by publicized cases? What are the consequences of such media attention—all too often inadequately informed? When is experimental therapy justified as an alternative option?[91]

Conclusions

Best interests is not really about law, or medicine. It is about everyone feeling that the best possible decision for a most vulnerable third party—a sick child—has been made. Enabling the right tone and mode of communication, which allows the identification of what is important for the individual child, her family, and wider societal implications, is crucial. For sure, advances in medicine lead us to believe (or want to believe) that life-sustaining treatment is a good thing. Yet the burdens of invasive critical care treatment cannot be underestimated. Once again, as in so many areas of medicine, communication between patients, their families, and the treating team is at the core of a positive experience even when the prognosis and ultimate outcomes are bleak. It is also crucial that all protagonists share the same interpretation of the child's interests, the potential for including consideration of what the child may want, and the possible scope of substituted decision making. Early intervention in conflict management is helpful and a mode of communication that enables views to be expressed and *heard* is necessary. Best interests is a useful concept and one which in the majority of cases serves us well, without ever having to get to a court of law. Nevertheless, development into a 'not against the child's interests' test may help to alleviate the perception that there is only one right answer. The adoption of a harm and benefits balance sheet is to be recommended as both a clinical exercise and an educative tool for parents of sick children, but only provided that the respective weight of the components is agreed and understood by all. Greater use of mediation or ethics committees in one guise or another may assist with this. In the long run, effective mediation and dispute resolution between parties would be far less costly (not only in financial terms but also emotional and reputational contexts).[92] Inevitably, as technology advances, more hard choices both as to cessation of treatment and the use of experimental treatment, need to be taken. Parents, as primary carers for their child, naturally want to take decisions regarding the child's treatment. The medical team as guardians of life and health logically want to do their best for the child's well-being. A focus on the child should normally mean that both perspectives come to the same conclusion. When this focus is lost, it is the role of the legal concept of best interests—including consideration of harm and what is not against the child's interests—that must decide the final outcome. Adult patients may have become 'entitled citizens',[93] but we should not forget that children, especially critically ill young children, need to have treatment decisions made for them. How the decision is made is just as important as who makes the decision itself.

References

1. In the UK, there is no legal distinction between withholding or withdrawing life-sustaining treatment: *Airedale NHS Trust v Bland* [1993] 1 All ER 821.
2. See, for example, within a vast literature: J. Montgomery, Law and the demoralisation of medicine (2006) 26 *Legal Studies* 185–210 at 202; J. Bridgeman, The provision of healthcare to young and dependent children: the principles, concepts and utility of the Children Act 1989 (2017) 25 *Medical Law Review* 363–96; E. Close et al., Charlie Gard: in defence of the law (2018) 44 *Journal of Medical Ethics* 476–80; T.M. Pope, The best interests standard: both guide and limit to medical decision making on behalf of incapacitated patients (2011) 22 *Journal of Clinical Ethics* 134–8.
3. *An NHS Trust v MB and another* [2006] EWHC 507 (Fam) per Holman J at [109].
4. J. Brierley, J. Linthicum, A. Petros, Should religious beliefs be allowed to stonewall a secular approach to withdrawing and withholding treatment in children? (2013) 39 *Journal of Medical Ethics* 573–7.
5. V. Larcher, F. Craig, K. Bhogal et al., Royal College of Paediatrics and Child Health, Making decisions to limit treatment in life-limiting and life-threatening conditions in children: a framework for practice (2015) 100 *Arch Dis Child* (Suppl 2) s3–23. This guidance has received judicial approval in a number of cases.
6. For example, the cases of Alfie Evans (Who was Alfie Evans and what was the row over his treatment? BBC News, 28 April 2018, http://www.bbc.co.uk/news/uk-england-merseyside-43754949 [accessed 5 December 2019]), Charlie Gard (A case that changed everything? BBC News, 29 July 2017, https://www.bbc.co.uk/news/health-40644896 [accessed 5 December 2019]), and Isaiah Haastrup's parents announce death of 'brave baby boy', BBC News, 8 March 2018, https://www.bbc.co.uk/news/uk-england-london-43328153 [accessed 5 December 2019]).
7. See the exchanges between S. Wilkinson and J. Savaulesu in a number of publications, collated in Practical ethics: the ethics of treatment for Charlie Gard: resources for students/media, http://blog.practicalethics.ox.ac.uk/2017/07/the-ethics-of-treatment-for-charlie-gard-resources-for-studentsmedia (accessed 5 December 2019).

8. See, for example, *Re D (A child)* [2019] UKSC 42, where it was held by a majority of the Supreme Court that parental agreement to the confinement of a 17-year-old with impaired decision-making capacity did not have the effect of taking his circumstances out of the scope of deprivation of liberty. Although the accommodation was held to be in his best interests, the majority of the Supreme Court held that a parent cannot provide substituted consent on behalf of a 16–17-year-old who is confined, if they are either unable or unwilling to give consent.

9. As suggested by the Nuffield Council of Bioethics in its report *Children and clinical research: ethical issues* (2015), at 4.33, https://nuffieldbioethics.org/publications/children-and-clinical-research (accessed 5 December 2019).

10. *J v C* [1969] 1 All ER 788 at 824, per Lord MacDermott.

11. Parental responsibility (PR) is the legal mechanism under s3(1) Children Act (CA) 1989, which recognizes who can make a decision regarding a child's upbringing. All mothers have automatic PR and, when she is married or in a civil partnership, her partner will also have PR: s2 and s4 CA 1989. Others may acquire PR by agreement or court order, including a local authority when a care order or emergency protection order is in place: s33(3) and s44(4) CA 1989. See R. Probert, S. Gilmore, J. Herring (eds) *Responsible parents and parental responsibility* (Oxford, Hart, 2009).

12. General Medical Council, *Good medical practice* (General Medical Council, 2013), para 48.

13. *Tafida Raqeeb v Barts NHS Foundation Trust* [2019] EWHC 2530 (Fam), at [182].

14. *In the Matter of Ashya King (A Child)* [2014] EWHC 2964, at [31].

15. A. Bainham, *Children: the modern law* (Bristol: Jordan Publishing, 2005.

16. R. Hain, Voices of moral authority: parents, doctors and what will actually help (2018) 44(7) *Journal of Medical Ethics* 458–61.

17. For example, when a local authority applies for a care order: s31 Children Act 1989.

18. *R v Wagstaffe* (1868) 10 Cox Crim Cas 530.

19. *R v Harris* 23 BMLR 122 (1995), commentary by D. Brahams (1993) 342 *Lancet* 1189.

20. Section 2(7) Children Act 1989: 'Where more than one person has parental responsibility for a child, each of them may act alone and without the other (or others) in meeting that responsibility; but nothing in this Part shall be taken to affect the operation of any enactment which requires the consent of more than one person in a matter affecting the child.'

21. *Re R (a minor)* [1991] 4 All ER 177 per Lord Donaldson MR, at 184.

22. See notably the case of *Re J (Child's Religion and Circumcision)* (2000) 52 BMLR 82 concerning the request by the child's father for the boy to be circumcised against the mother's wishes. Butler Sloss LJ recognised that there were 'a small group

of important decisions which, in the absence of agreement of those with parental responsibility, ought not to be carried out or arranged by one-parent carer [...]. Such a decision ought not to be made without the specific approval of a court' [at 88].

23. Section 8(1) Family Law Reform Act 1969.

24. *Re D (A child)* [2019] UKSC 42, at [26(i)]. Pre-Human Rights Act case law proceeded on the basis that parents could do so: see *Re W (a minor)(medical treatment: court's jurisdiction)* [1993] Fam 64.

25. *Re P* [2014] EWHC 1650 (Fam).

26. Of course, this justification would fail in the case of a competent adult, so the decision begs the question whether, having found the adolescent to be competent, the court should legitimately invoke its inherent jurisdiction to decide on the best interests of the patient, or whether, in fact, the regime applicable to adults should by extension be applicable to competent 17-year-olds.

27. *Re D (A child)* [2019] UKSC 42 upholding an appeal from the decision of Munby, P in *Re D (A child)* [2017] EWCA Civ 1695.

28. See the so-called Fraser guidelines in *Gillick v West Norfolk & Wisbech AHA* (1986) AC 112, confirmed in *R(Axon) v Secretary of State for Health* [2006] EWCA 37 (Admin).

29. *Re E (a minor) (wardship:medical treatment)* [1993] 1 FLR 386; *Re W (a minor) (medical treatment: court's jurisdiction)* [1992] 1 FLR 1.

30. See, for example, Baker J in *A Local Health Board v Y (A Child) & Ors* [2016] EWHC 206 (Fam) where he noted that 'Putting myself in Y's position, and considering matters from his point of view, I conclude that, were he able to express his own wishes and feelings, he would accept that the course of treatment proposed by the clinicians is in his best interests', at [19].

31. See *An NHS Trust v SK (Best Interests Decision—Palliative Care)* [2016] EWHC 2860 (Fam) where the judge expressly refers to the 'assumed point of view' of the 11-year-old and explicitly rejects the mother's perspective, which was found to be overly burdensome (at [54]).

32. However, when a local authority exercises PR, even if in agreement with the proposed treatment, recourse to the court is recommended: *Re SE* [2014] EWHC 3182 (Fam).

33. As originally suggested in *Airedale NHS Trust v Bland* [1993] AC 789.

34. *An NHS Trust and others v Y (by his litigation friend the Official Solicitor) and another* [2018] UKSC 46.

35. *Re A (conjoined twins)* [2000] EWCA Civ 254 per Ward LJ, at [14].

36. General Medical Council, *Treatment and care towards the end of life: good practice in decision making* (General Medical Council, 2010), para 108. https://www.gmc-uk.org/-/media/documents/treatment-and-care-towards-the-

end-of-life---english-1015_pdf-48902105.pdf?la=en&hash=41EF651C76FDBE C141FB674C08261661BDEFD004 (accessed 5 December 2019).

37. *Glass v UK* [2004] 1 FLR 1019; *Tafida Raqeeb v Barts NHS Foundation Trust* [2019] EWHC 2530 (Fam), at [114].

38. On the relevance of using the Children Act orders, instead of the wider inherent jurisdiction of the court, see the insightful analysis by J. Bridgeman, The provision of healthcare to young and dependent children: the principles, concepts, and utility of the Children act 1989 (2017) 25 *Medical Law Review* 363–396.

39. *Re E (a child)* [2018] EWCA Civ 550, [at 93–94].

40. *Re OT (a child)* [2009] EWCA Civ 409.

41. Citing *Portsmouth Hospital NHS Trust v Wyatt* [2005] 1 WLR 3995, at [98].

42. *Gard and others v UK* Appl. 39793/17, 27th June 2017.

43. *Portsmouth Hospital NHS Trust v Wyatt* [2004] EWHC. 2247, at [4].

44. *R (Burke) v General Medical Council* [2005] EWCA Civ 1003.

45. Nor, unless the doctor was acting entirely irrationally, could thecourts cannot *order* a doctor to continue treatment: see *An NHS Trust v MB (2006)* EWHC 507 (Fam) per Holman J, at [90]; and *St George's Healthcare NHS Trust v P* [2015] EWCOP 42, where despite 'ordering and directing treatment to continue' the declaration simply declared lawful the continued treatment of the patient.

46. *Re B (adult: refusal of medical treatment)* [2002] 2 All ER 449.

47. *Aintree University Hospitals NHS Foundation Trust v James and others* [2013] UKSC 67, at [22].

48. *Re E (a child)* [2018] EWCA Civ 550; *Re A* [2016] EWCA Civ 759.

49. Per Lady Hale in *Aintree*, at [39].

50. See, for example, *A Local Health Board v Y (A Child) & Ors* [2016] EWHC 206 (Fam) and *An NHS Trust v SK (Best Interests Decision—Palliative Care)* [2016] EWHC 2860 (Fam).

51. *Re R (A minor) (Wardship: consent to treatment)* [1992] Fam 11 per Lord Donaldson MR.

52. Holman J in *An NHS Trust v. MB* [2006] 2 FLR 319.

53. *Tafida Raqeeb v Barts NHS Foundation Trust* [2019] EWHC 2530 (Fam), at [191].

54. Ibid, at [122].

55. *Re A (a child)* [2016] EWCA Civ 759, at [58].

56. *Tafida Raqeeb v Barts NHS Foundation Trust* [2019] EWHC 2530 (Fam), at [168].

57. *Re J* [1990] 3 All ER 930 per Balcome LJ [at 938]. In this case, Taylor J suggested that the test could be whether the child 'if capable of exercising sound judgment would consider life tolerable', at 945.

58. *Re T (a minor) (Wardship: medical treatment)* per Waite LJ (1997) 1 WLR 242, at 253.

59. *Re A (Male Sterilisation)* [2000] 1 FLR 549, per Butler Sloss LJ, at [555].

60. M. Donnelly, Best interests in the Mental Capacity Act—time to say goodbye? (2016) 24(3) *Medical Law Review* 318–32.

61. Tom L. Beauchamp, James F. Childress, *Principles of biomedical ethics*, 5th edition (New York: Oxford University Press, 2001), pp. 99–103.

62. *A (A Child), Re* [2016] EWCA Civ 759, at [56]. A good example of a balance sheet, and awareness that alone it cannot reflect the preponderate weight of the different elements, can be found in *Re MB* [2006] EWHC 507 (Fam).

63. *Re E (a minor) (wardship: medical treatment)*(1992) 9 BMLR 1.

64. Ibid; also *Re P* [2014] EWHC 1650 (Fam).

65. *Re T (a minor) (Wardship: medical treatment)* [1997] 1 FLR 502, confirmed in *Re MB* [2006] EWHC 507 (Fam).

66. A classic example would be the decision that it was in an incompetent adult's best interests to donate bone marrow to their sibling: *Re Y (mental incapacity)*[1996] 2 FLR 787.

67. *Re MB* [2006] EWHC 507 (Fam), at para 64–6.

68. G. Birchley, Deciding together? Best interests and shared decision-making in paediatric intensive care (2014) 22 *Health Care Analysis* 203–22.

69. R. Gillon, Why Charlie Gard's parents should have been the decision makers about their son's best interests (2018) 44 *Journal of Medical Ethics*, 462–5.

70. Permission decision in the case of Charlie Gard, 19 June 2017, UKSC at [17].

71. For an analysis of how the harm principle might apply in practice, see D. Diekema, Parental refusals of medical treatment: the harm principle as threshold for state intervention (2004) 25 *Theoretical Medicine*, 243–64.

72. Section 31 Children Act 1989.

73. [2017] EWHC 972 (Fam) at [49].

74. On this point, see J. Bridgman, A threshold of significant harm (f)or a viable alternative therapeutic option (2018) 44 *Journal of Medical Ethics* 466–70.

75. *Re E (a child)* [2018] EWCA Civ 550.

76. Ibid., at [111].

77. G. Birchley, Harm is all you need? Best interests and disputes about parental decision-making (2016) 42 *Journal of Medical Ethics* 111–15.

78. J. Bridgeman, *Gard and Yates v GOSH, the Guardian and the UK*: reflections on the legal process and the legal principles (2017) 17(4) *Medical Law International* 285–302.

79. *Affaire Marwa, Conseil d'Etat*, 8 March 2017, Assistance Publique—Hôpitaux de Marseille, n° 408146.

80. See, for example, L. Marguet, Entre protection objective et conception subjective…(2017) *La Revue des Droits de l'Homme*, http://journals.openedition.org/revdh/2866 (accessed 5 December 2019), and C. Bourdaire-Mignot, T. Grundler, Le médecin, les parents et le juge. Trois regards sur l'obstination déraisonnable

(2017) *La Revue des Droits de l'Homme*, Actualités Droits-Libertés, https://journals.openedition.org/revdh/3050 (accessed 5 December 2019).

81. But such an approach may fall foul to claims of paternalism, as some have suggested is the consequence of not requiring a court declaration to withdraw treatment from an adult when the parties are in agreement: C. Foster, The rebirth of medical paternalism: an NHS Trust v Y (2018) *Journal of Medical Ethics*, published online first: 9 October 2018.

82. R. Huxtable, Clinic, courtroom or (specialist) committee—in the best interests of the critically ill child? (2018) 44 *Journal of Medical Ethics* 471–5. In the US, all hospitals provide a clinical ethics consultation service.

83. R. Hain, Voices of moral authority: parents, doctors and what will actually help (2018) 44(7) *Journal of Medical Ethics* 458–61. However, the legal foundation of such a panel would be dubious. Unless the parties agreed to be bound by it—for example, by analogy with arbitration—then it could not be constitutionally recognized in the same way as a tribunal or court.

84. Close et al., Charlie Gard; C. Wallis, When paediatricians and families can't agree (2018) 103 *Arch Dis Child* 413–14.

85. *Great Ormond Street Hospital for Children NHS Foundation Trust v Yates and others* [2017] EWHC 972 (Fam) [at 130].

86. Great Ormond Street Hospital for Children NHS Foundation Trust, *1st clinical ethics service report: the child first and always* (GOSH, 2015).

87. S. Meller, S. Barclay, Mediation: an approach to intractable disputes between parents and paediatricians (2011) 96 *Arch Dis Child* 619–21, at 619.

88. L. Forbat, S. Barclay, Reducing healthcare conflict: outcomes from using the conflict management framework (2018) *Archives of Disease in Childhood*, published online first: 28 August, doi: 10.1136/archdischild-2018-315647 (accessed 5 December 2019).

89. Medicines for Human Use (Clinical Trials) Regulations 2004.

90. Royal College of Paediatrics, Child Health, Ethics Advisory Committee, Guidelines for the ethical conduct of medical research involving children (2000) *82 Arch Disease in Childhood* 177–82.

91. It is interesting to note a declaration that experimental stem cell therapy was in an incapacitous adult's best interests insofar as it was important psychologically to give effect to their wish to try the therapy: *Re D (Medical Treatment)* [2017] EWCOP 15.

92. See the model proposed in D. Wilkinson, S. Barclay, J. Savulescu, Disagreement, mediation, arbitration: resolving disputes about medical treatment (2018) 391 *Lancet* 2302–5.

93. J. Montgomery, Patient no longer? What next in healthcare law? (2017) 70 *Current Legal Problems* 73–109.

5

Adults Who Lack Capacity to Consent and Deprivation of Liberty

Daniele Bryden

Introduction to incapacity

The complexities of consent within the intensive care environment have been discussed in Chapter 1. Irrespective of those difficulties, it remains a fundamental principle of UK medical ethics to recognize an individual's right to autonomy and self-determination. However, differing views as to the nature of autonomy exist from one of simple independence of decision making to those that encompass a need to incorporate additional values such as an ability to form goals based on initial desires and wishes.[1]

This chapter will first consider the historical common law position of capacity and then discuss the implications of statutory developments—namely, the Adults with Incapacity (Scotland) Act 2000 and the Mental Capacity Act 2005 (MCA).

Prior to the legislative definitions of capacity, common law presumed an adult's competence to make decisions and protected a patient's right to give or withhold consent irrespective of their reasoning behind the decision. There was arguably a more nuanced view of autonomy because the patient was required to display rational thinking.[2] The patient also needed to understand the clinician's proposal, something outside the clinician's direct control. All health professionals still need to provide sufficient information to patients to enable them to attempt to make a decision. However, an additional factor is the multi-cultural, multi-linguistic nature of the UK patient population, which brings into question additional concerns regarding comprehension. As an example, understanding of the term 'unconscious' was shown to be poor in a sample of 700 individuals, and worse for those who do not have English as a first language.[3]

However, the law is concerned principally with the manner of disclosure so that information is given in a way that is capable of being understood.

As already outlined, consent is a process of information exchange between health professional and patient that allows a patient to exercise their right to autonomy. As such, it is equally valid for a patient to refuse information providing she is aware of her entitlement to it, although the Code of Practice for the Adults with Incapacity (Scotland) Act counsels professionals to watch out for undue influence from others on a patient and their decisions regarding consent.[4] Intensive care decision making is often conducted in a time frame where consent can only infrequently be considered to be a process, and where many patients for various reasons do not retain capacity.

This chapter will consider how issues such as consent and capacity apply to critical care practice and how considerations in cases of incapacity such as the 'best interests' and 'substituted judgements' tests are considered. It will also examine the changes that have occurred in relation to the law on deprivation of liberty and how the courts and Law Commission have recognized the unique nature of the environment in which care is provided.

Development of best interests test

It is a general common law principle that unauthorized contact between individuals is criminal assault, unless it falls under one of the recognized exceptions vitiated by consent and discussed by the House of Lords in *R v Brown*.[5] Moreover, unauthorized touching could also constitute a civil tort, delict of battery, or trespass. In the case of Ms B, who continued to receive life-sustaining ventilation despite her wishes to the contrary, she was awarded nominal damages for the tort recognizing that 'there is a serious danger of a benevolent paternalism which does not embrace recognition of the personal autonomy of the severely disabled patient'.[6] For the law to uphold these principles in the face of a severely ill or injured patient needing life-saving treatment in intensive care would be nonsense, and section 5 of the Mental Capacity Act 2005 requires an individual to take 'reasonable steps to establish whether [the person] lacks capacity in relation to the matter in question, and ... that it will be in [the person's] best interests for the act to be done'.

In order for a proposed course of action to be lawful within the context of the Mental Capacity Act, it must not just be a matter of convenience to do so without waiting for the patient to recover capacity—for example, the intensive care patient who has an acute airway problem requiring intubation and mechanical ventilation may well progress on to receiving a tracheostomy to facilitate their ongoing care and reduce any further risks to their person. If it is reasonably possible to delay any treatment until the patient regains capacity, that should be the case regardless of whether there may be an additional medical benefit to the patient.[7] This might apply to the incidental finding of an additional medical condition that is not life threatening and does not affect the course of the patient's treatment on the intensive care unit (ICU)—for example, the presence of an ovarian cyst seen on CT scan images of the abdomen performed to assess the extent of pelvic trauma. In *Williamson v East London HA*, a patient underwent a mastectomy without consent having agreed only to the removal of a leaking breast implant.[8] The court found for the patient because, although the operation would have been necessary at some point, she had not had this possibility discussed with her and would not have given her consent then had it been discussed with her.

Section 4 of the MCA requires healthcare staff to try to obtain information from any family member or friend if a patient is unconscious 'to discover any anticipatory choice on the part of the patient or other details which might affect a clinical decision'.[9] Although a statutory requirement to try and establish this, because of the emergency and unanticipated nature of many ICU admissions, it is more common for patients to have made no prior declaration as to their wishes and so this rarely forms the sole basis by which treatment decisions are made.

The difficulty for critical care professionals is that there are often intercurrent conditions in our patient population such as pain, hypoxia, sepsis, etc. which can often bring into doubt any adult's capacity to make decisions regarding life-saving treatments. Physical pain and emotional distress have been identified as vitiating factors in negating the ability of a pregnant woman to weigh up adequately the considerations necessary in her refusal to undergo a forceps delivery.[10] Historically, the gravity and potential for such treatments to be literally life-saving might have suggested that less evidence was needed to rebut any presumption of competence. 'The graver the consequences of the decision, the commensurately greater the level of competence is required to take the decision'.[11] However, the recent case of *Kings College NHS Foundation Trust v C and V* casts doubt on whether that view is still the case.[12] Mrs C's ongoing refusal to undergo renal dialysis, despite the fact that it would lead to her death, was considered by MacDonald J to be an 'unwise' one. Nevertheless, he held that:

> C has capacity to decide whether or not to accept treatment. C is entitled to make her own decision on that question based on the things that are important to her, in keeping with her own personality and system of values and without conforming to society's expectation of what constitutes the 'normal' decision in this situation (if such a thing exists). As a capacitous individual C is, in respect of her own body and mind, sovereign.

MacDonald J has outlined the difficulties of identifying an individual's 'best interests' when in effect a normative standard is being applied. In *Re F*, concerning a proposal to sterilize a mentally handicapped woman deemed incapable of making a competent decision regarding the procedure, Lord Goff recognized the problems for professionals working in more acute areas, and suggested that 'the doctor must act in accordance with a responsible and competent body of relevant professional opinion, on the principles set down in *Bolam v Friern Hospital Management Committee*'.[13] Therefore, until the introduction of the Mental Capacity Act 2005, it was left to professional medical opinion to determine what was in the patient's best interests with accusations of paternalism, and confusion over the narrowness or breadth of 'best interests'. Subsequent examinations of the test in cases like *Airedale NHS Trust v Bland*[14] and *Re MB*[15] have considered best interests to be much wider considerations than the purely medical: Butler-Sloss LJ's view summarizes this as 'best interests encompasses medical, emotional and all other welfare issues'.[16] However, the 'Bolam' test is not always sufficient to judge best interests[17] and the ultimate decision will rest with the courts.[18]

The problems with considerations of best interests and its subsequent examination by bodies such as the Law Commission led to the creation of the Mental Capacity Act 2005 in England and Wales, following on from the Adults with Incapacity (Scotland) Act 2000.

Intensive care practitioners in England and Wales now operate in an environment where there is a statutory definition of 'best interests'. Section 4 of the MCA determines best interests in the context of provision of life-sustaining treatment as one where an individual 'must not, in considering whether the treatment is in the best interests of the person concerned, be motivated by a desire to bring about his death'. He or she must consider:

(6) (a) the person's past and present wishes and feelings (and, in particular, any relevant written statement made by him when he had capacity),
　(b) the beliefs and values that would be likely to influence his decision if he had capacity, and
　(c) the other factors that he would be likely to consider if he were able to do so.
(7) He must take into account, if it is practicable and appropriate to consult them, the views of—
　(a) anyone named by the person as someone to be consulted on the matter in question or on matters of that kind,
　(b) anyone engaged in caring for the person or interested in his welfare,

(c) any donee of a lasting power of attorney granted by the person, and

(d) any deputy appointed for the person by the court, as to what would be in the person's best interests ...

Many of the treatments provided within the intensive care environment fall under the definition of 'Life-sustaining treatment' as treatment 'which in the view of a person providing health care for the person concerned is necessary to sustain life.'

Section 2 of the Mental Capacity Act defines incapacity as when 'a person lacks capacity in relation to a matter if at the material time he is unable to make a decision for himself in relation to the matter because of an impairment of, or a disturbance in the functioning of, the mind or brain'. Along with the section 3(1) requirements to understand the relevant information, retain it, use it as part of the decision-making process and communicate the decision, it clarifies some of these difficulties for critical care professionals who must regularly make decisions regarding the wisdom of initiating treatment in incapacitated adults. It can be less clear, however, how healthcare professionals should utilize the 'best interests' test when treatments are already established.

In relation to provision of treatment at the end of life, the General Medical Council (GMC), regulator for all doctors within the UK, counsels providing or withdrawing treatments on the basis of what is of 'overall benefit' to the individual.[19] This is an unusual term not identified in either statute but could be considered as an attempt by the GMC to capture the concepts of 'best interests' and benefits of treatment operating across all UK legislations.

Substituted judgement test

In contrast, the substituted judgement test is more widely used for considerations of treatment of the incompetent patient in the USA. It tries to second guess what a patient would have chosen in a particular set of circumstances in contrast to the best interests test that uses information to try to decide what on balance is best for that patient. At first glance, it would seem to be a more subjective assessment, and less paternalistic than the best interests test. However, it is often the case that an incapacitated patient on the ICU cannot express any sort of choice, and has rarely had previous experience of the proposed treatment requiring a decision—for example, tracheostomy to facilitate weaning. In effect, the ICU doctor would look to a third party, whether relative or other colleague with previous clinical responsibility for the patient, to substitute the patient's decision. Therefore, in practice, the third party is using their *own* judgement to second guess that of the patient's based on what they know of their prior expressed thoughts and behaviours. This is subject to heavy criticism as flawed and 'in the absence of real evidence equivalent to guesswork'.[20] It is interesting that the test has been applied to the case of Nancy Cruzan in the USA, where an application was sought to remove artificial nutrition and hydration from her while she existed in a permanent vegetative state. The court did demand the need for evidence that not continuing to exist in a vegetative state was consistent with Nancy's wishes, and this was able to be provided by both her friends and parents. The US courts appear to have adopted a position that, in using the substituted judgement test, the presumption is to adopt continuation of life-preserving treatment as a default position because this causes less harm to the incompetent individual.

As commentators like McLean have noted, use of a substituted judgement test is often very difficult to apply and as open to abuse as the best interests test. Harm may equally well come from being kept alive in a state with no prospect of recovery, or in such a way that assumes that the individual would not have had any interests in how they were cared for, or without considering the possibility that parties who are consulted will have their own interests in the outcome:

> Close family members may have a strong feeling … that they do not wish to witness the continuation of the life of a loved one which they regard as hopeless … there is no automatic assurance that the view of close family members will necessarily be the same as the patient's would have been had she been confronted with the prospect of her situation.[21]

Overlap of best interests and substituted judgement

At a basic level, healthcare practitioners working within critical care environments routinely attempt to establish a patient's views on their treatments and likely future health desires as part of good practice standards. However, this is only in relation to the extent of any treatment that is consistent with professional judgement and not as a way of enforcing treatment that is not considered medically appropriate.[22]

While the substituted judgement test is not directly accepted, in practice some consideration is given to the postulated wishes of the incompetent patient. At issue, however, is often the degree to which emphasis is given to these 'estimated wishes'. The recent case of David James has arguably pushed the position in England and Wales nearer to a substituted judgement test. Mr James was a patient on an ICU who had suffered a stroke, cardiac arrest and was at least partially dependent on a ventilator to assist his breathing. He was significantly neurologically impaired and lacked capacity to make decisions about his own medical treatment. Nonetheless, there was some evidence of him getting pleasure from family interaction. The medical opinion was that he was unlikely ever to leave the critical care unit, let alone the hospital. The hospital wished to limit the degree of intensive care treatments—for example, cardiovascular and renal support he would receive if he were to deteriorate further. The family opposed this.

The Supreme Court supported an earlier Court of Appeal decision to give the hospital permission on the basis that 'the focus is on whether it is in the patient's best interests to give the treatment, rather than on whether it is in his best interests to withhold or withdraw it.'[23] The best interests test is wide, encompassing a holistic assessment, 'not just medical but social and psychological'.

It is arguable that in clinical practice there may be very little difference (if any now) between the best interests and substituted judgement tests when considering a patient who lacks capacity. In *Salford Royal NHS Foundation Trust v Mrs P & Anor*, the Trust sought a declaration to continue clinically assisted artificial nutrition and hydration in an individual who was in a minimally conscious state. The application was refused and the evidence given by the family as to her wishes was influential:

> [The Patient's] present high level of dependency and minimal awareness would, to her, have been 'a travesty of life', to adopt her own phase. Many other people have wholly different views; [the Patient] is entitled to hers. Her incapacitous state does not mean her wishes can be disregarded. Her family, each of them, has permitted her voice to be heard and thus enabled her to assert her own autonomy.[24]

Because, as part of the statutory definition of 'best interests', the Mental Capacity Act requires consultation with individuals in the absence of an advance decision, it is likely that these individuals may either have a good idea of the incompetent person's wishes or have been given specific instructions. In both situations, therefore, consultation using best interests guidance is arguably a more formalized version of the substituted judgement test, particularly within UK ICU practice where it is an almost universal practice to obtain information from relatives or carers as to any known prior wishes expressed by the patient.

In David James's case, Lady Hale noted that the decision maker:

> must consider, so far as is reasonably ascertainable (a) the person's past and present wishes and feelings (and, in particular, any relevant written statement made by him when he had capacity) (b) the beliefs and values that would be likely to influence his decision if he had capacity, and (c) the other factors that he would be likely to consider if he were able to do so.

On the face of it, the test remains one of best interests, 'but one which accepts that the preferences of the person concerned are an important component in deciding where his best interests lie'. This looks very close to substituted judgement but on an uncertain basis. Is it the judgement of the person as they were when they were healthy or looking at the person as they are now? The two are ethically very different. There is ample evidence to suggest that, when we are in the situation we have most devoutly feared, we are far more able to bear it than we thought we would be. When much is stripped from us, we value all the more what is left.[25]

Temporary incapacity

Treatment decisions

On an ICU, it is more usual to encounter patients who lack capacity on a temporary basis due to illness, drugs, or hypoxia. It is not unusual, therefore, for healthcare professionals to arguably adopt a 'default' presumption of incapacity rather than to assume the required position of capacity for decision making. Much of the case law concerning incapacity relates to patients who have a relatively long-term lack of capacity—for example, learning disability where the issue is one of whether the individual is competent to make a particular decision such as sterilization. However, in the critical care population, lack of capacity is often less open to dispute: many patients are unconscious or sedated, but this may be temporary and the issues relate to the appropriateness of a decision in those circumstances where capacity may be regained at a later point or, in some individuals, never regained at all.

The vast majority of decisions about incapacitated adults are taken by carers and others without any formal general authority because there is no automatic proxy consent for another person.[26] Although it is generally considered good practice to inform a patient's 'next of kin'[a] of any plans to perform surgery,

---

[a] 'A category that has no formal legal status, contrary to popular (and often clinical belief.'

this does not constitute a process of consent. Such conversations may be very useful in informing the doctor's decision, but it is inappropriate to ask relatives to sign a 'consent' form. Section 5 of the Mental Capacity Act has created a statutory defence for all healthcare professionals who treat an incapacitated adult, provided they have a reasonable belief that the act is in the person's best interests.[27]

Similarly, forms that are used to document such decisions are not consent forms but rather a means to record that the procedure is being carried out in a collaborative way, and to allow staff to formally record and consider the necessity of any treatment at such a point. Section 6 of the Mental Capacity Act now also provides a lawful means to provide restraint to facilitate treatment when this does not shade into deprivation of liberty (see further below). While this may seem paternalistic, the assumption is that the intervention is probably necessary to allow the patient to recover to such a point where they can form their own decision—for example, holding an oxygen mask on a confused patient who may become less confused as their oxygenation improves.

Deprivation of liberty

Deprivation of Liberty Safeguards (DoLS) were introduced in April 2009 allied to the Mental Capacity Act 2005 to provide a legislative template allowing individuals in a registered setting such as a care home or hospital to have their deprivation of liberty considered and, if appropriate, authorized in compliance with the Article 5 right to liberty and freedom of the person outlined in the European Convention on Human Rights and the Human Rights Act 1998. While intended to provide objective assessment and protection for individuals who do not have capacity—for example, those with dementia—other individuals like intensive care patients were considered to have been 'caught up' in its application. This was identified by Lady Hale in the Supreme Court in relation to a case commonly known as 'Cheshire West' whereby three individuals unable to consent to their community care, which on occasion required use of physical or chemical restraint, were determined to have been deprived of their liberty. The 'acid test' for a deprivation of liberty outlined by Lady Hale was that of 'continuous supervision and control and not free to leave'.[28] The apparent applicability of this scope to intensive care practice resulted in considerable uncertainty for intensive care practitioners and hospitals, which led to a ten-fold increase in the number of applications to local authorities from hospitals for authorization of deprivations of liberty apparently arising from medical treatment.[29]

The subsequent case of Maria Ferreira has helped to clarify the current case law in relation to deprivation of liberty and receipt of medical treatment on an ICU. Maria Ferreira had Down's syndrome and was unable to consent to her medical treatment on the ICU from which she unfortunately did not recover. Her sister had brought judicial review proceedings against the coroner, arguing that Maria's death had occurred in state detention because her liberty had been deprived while in the ICU. The initial application was dismissed and a subsequent hearing at the Court of Appeal provided necessary clarity for treatment within an intensive care setting. Arden LJ, giving judgment, identified specific authorized exceptions from Article 5(1) of the European Convention on Human Rights, which included 'any deprivation of liberty resulting from the administration of life-saving treatment'. Moreover ... 'treatment must be given in good faith and is materially the same treatment as would be given to a person of sound mind with the same physical illness' (paragraph 93).

As a result of this judgment, there is likely to be no deprivation of liberty where a patient is unable to leave the hospital as a result of their medical condition or its treatment, rather than any restrictions imposed by the hospital staff—for example, continuous nursing supervision, or use of medication. Therefore, where treatment is being administered in these circumstances, the requirement for authorization under DoLS does not apply.

Disputes regarding capacity or best interests that cannot be resolved locally—for example, disputes between family and treating teams regarding prognosis and ongoing treatment—may need to be resolved by involving second opinions, considering mediation, or, ultimately, by application to the Court of Protection.

A 2017 review into DoLS safeguards by the Law Commission in 2017 criticized them for being overly complicated and bureaucratic, and there was evidence (not just in intensive care practice) that people were not actively engaged in the processor placing appropriate weight on any evidence of prior wishes.[30]

In July 2018, the UK Government introduced a draft Bill, the Mental Capacity (Amendment) Bill,[31] to address some of these issues. The Law Commission's proposed reforms going beyond considerations of deprivation of liberty to impose a change from a passive duty to consider the wishes and feelings of an individual to an active duty to ascertain them. These were not introduced in the Bill, which was narrowly focused on reforms to the process of authorization of deprivation of liberty, intended to be less burdensome to stakeholders, speed up the process of assessment and consider restrictions of a person's liberty as part of their overall care package. The Government's intention was for there to be a statutory definition of deprivation of liberty but, at the time of writing, Parliament was divided on whether one should be introduced. It remains to be determined whether those receiving treatment on intensive care, and deprived of their capacity and liberty by nature of their illness and necessary treatment, will once again be inadvertently caught up in the considerations of any future iterations of this Bill.

Other considerations in temporary incapacity

There are, however, instances when a patient may be rendered temporarily incapacitated on an ICU, and when there are requests from police officers to perform tests or take samples to facilitate a criminal investigation. This can often lead to confusion among healthcare staff as to the conflicts between the need to protect patient confidentiality and the requirements of the law when a patient is incapacitated.

The Human Tissue Act 2004 concerns requests for DNA samples and identifies any removal of human tissue without consent (including blood and skin cells) as an offence unless the action falls within a list of excepted purposes such as to facilitate the functions of a coroner, or to investigate or prosecute a crime.

Doctors have an ethical duty to protect patient confidentiality, but this may come into conflict with a requirement on us, as for any member of society, not to impede a criminal investigation. Staff caring for a patient who has been involved in a road traffic collision may be approached if there are genuine police concerns that drugs or alcohol were involved in the event. Under those circumstances, introducing a time delay to wait for the patient to regain capacity may result in the loss of important evidence. The Police Reform Act 2002 allows for samples to be taken without waiting for recovery of capacity, although testing of the specimen is not allowed until the patient recovers capacity and, having been informed by the police officer that a sample has been taken, gives agreement for the sample to be used in this way. Healthcare professionals are in a position to object to the sample being taken, but only if the sampling process hinders patient care. If the specimen is not necessary for the patient's care, but the Police Reform Act requires it, it would be better, if time allows, to get someone appropriately trained but not involved in patient care, such as a police surgeon or another staff member, to take the sample, to avoid this conflict of interest.

Other forms of testing, such as HIV testing, may be part of specific professional guidance from bodies like the GMC, which recommends non-consensual testing if it is in the patient's best interests. The recent case of the Skripals, victims of presumed Novichok poisoning, confirmed this view. Sedated on an ICU and unable to consent to further testing, disclosure of their medical records to experts from the Organisation for the Prohibition of Chemical Weapons (OPCW) was considered lawful by Mr Justice Williams on the basis that 'there may be some potential medical benefit in the tests being conducted by the OPCW in that they may identify some matter which sheds further light on the nature of the agent involved and thus the treatment that might be administered,'[32] as well as on the basis that, were the Skripals at that point in a position to express a view, they would want steps to be taken to enable the rule of law to be upheld.

While testing among those thought to be at risk of many treatable viral conditions is recommended during a hospital admission, it should be possible to wait until the patient recovers capacity for many of these tests unless clinically indicated. It is not automatically always appropriate to conduct these tests during the ICU phase of an admission. In certain circumstances and where clinically indicated, such as part of a non-invasive liver screen, it is appropriate to test while a person is incapacitated on the ICU. Medical staff, however, do not receive exemptions to allow testing of an unconscious patient if they suffer a blood borne virus incident while at work. Samples can be taken but cannot be tested until the patient recovers capacity to consent.

Permanent incapacity from unconsciousness

However, some patients may never recover consciousness, so entering into a process of consent is impossible and there is no utility from delays in treatment providing the treatment can be shown to be in their best interests. There can, of course, be considerable difficulty in determining where those best interests may lie.

This is exemplified by the case of Anthony Bland, a young man who had been left in a permanent vegetative state following a hypoxic cerebral injury he sustained during the Hillsborough stadium crowd disaster.[33]

Anthony Bland's life was sustained in part by artificial enteral feeding and both his family and the medical team caring for him were of the view that it was inappropriate to continue feeding him in this manner. Airedale NHS Trust therefore sought a declaration that they could lawfully discontinue this feeding, which was challenged by the Official Solicitor as a proposed course of action amounting to unlawful killing. The first instance decision included a judgment from Sir Stephen Brown that withdrawal of feeding was consistent with Anthony's best interests having 'no therapeutic, medical or other benefit … in continuing to maintain his ventilation, nutrition and hydration by artificial means'. The same test was supported by the Court of Appeal, with an extension of reasoning to include consideration of the 'constant invasions and humiliations' his body was subjected to from the treatment, the effects these would have on previous memories of him, the 'prolonged ordeal imposed on all members of his family', and also an altruistic notion that 'finite resources are better devoted to enhancing life than simply averting death'.

The House of Lords' view as to the application of the best interests test in Bland's case was controversial in that it was held that 'the proposed conduct is not in the best interests of Anthony Bland, for he has no best interests of any kind'.[34] In their Lordships' view, it was meaningless to apply the best interests test to the permanently unconscious, and continuation or withdrawal of further treatment should not be decided using the test. Rather, they took the view that the best interests test should be reversed and consideration given to the utility of continuing with treatment that artificially prolongs life with an obligation on medical staff to stop further treatment:

> If there comes a stage where the responsible doctor comes to the reasonable conclusion (which accords with the views of a responsible body of medical opinion) that further continuance of an intrusive life support system is not in the best interests of the patient, he can no longer lawfully continue that life support system: to do so would constitute the crime of battery and the tort of trespass to the person.

This is not an isolated decision because the Inner House of the Court of session in Scotland took the same view—that, in cases of permanent unconsciousness, the correct application of the best interests test was a negative one, and that there could be no interest in being kept alive by artificial means.[35]

What then of cases where there are differences in medical opinion? In the case of Bland, Lord Browne-Wilkinson took the view that the application to the courts to discontinue life-prolonging treatment would be supported if there was a reasonable body of medical opinion, and that this was not negated by the presence of an opposing medical viewpoint: 'the courts' only concern will be to be satisfied that the doctors' decision to discontinue is in accordance with a respectable body of medical opinion that it is reasonable'.[36]

This would appear to be legal support for a paternalistic view of medical care that does not make full use of the best interests test, whether because, as some have argued, the view that permanent unconsciousness can have only a negative application of the best interests test is not making full use of the test,[37] or rather that the test in such cases should be replaced by the substituted judgement test as being ethically preferable.[38]

Determining best interests post Mental Capacity Act 2005

Both *Aintree* and *Re Y* have now established that the best interests considerations of the Mental Capacity Act apply in cases of permanent loss of previously capacitous individuals. The British Medical Association has also produced guidance for medical practitioners regarding the use and withdrawal of artificial nutrition and hydration to that effect.[39] It has been considered by Dame Butler-Sloss in the light of the Human Rights Act 1998 and is not held to be a contravention of an Article 2 Right to life.[40] Denzil Lush (Master of the Court of Protection) has argued that the MCA has moved the best interests test nearer to the substituted judgement test because there is an obligation for health professionals to consult.[41] Similarly, by using the language of Bolam in the House of Lords, there is a suggestion that actions like treatment withdrawal must be supportable by peer professional opinion. While there was no obligation in Lord Browne-Wilkinson's judgment to obtain peer opinion, it would seem reasonable that doctors within critical care who consult and canvass additional opinions will be in a better position to support decisions as to withdrawals of treatment in the unconscious patient when the options are continuing treatment with no prospect of making the patient fit enough to recover capacity or to withdraw treatment that is needlessly prolonging life. This is firmly established in *re Y* that in cases of:

> a lack of agreement to a proposed course of action from those with an interest in the patient's welfare, a court application can and should be made ... approaching a court in the event of doubts as to the best interests of the patient is an essential part of the protection of human rights. The assessments, evaluations and opinions assembled as part of the medical process will then form the core of the material available to the judge, together with such further expert and other evidence as may need to be placed before the court at that stage.

Treatment which is of no direct benefit

There are difficulties in relation to the incompetent adult receiving treatment on an ICU that has no direct bearing on the course of their present condition. In the case of Stephen Blood, a man who died after receiving treatment on an ICU for meningitis, the issue was in relation to treatment he received on the ICU to obtain sperm samples prior to his death, when his consent for the procedure was impossible to obtain. Subsequent use of the sperm was contrary to the requirement to have written permission from the donor as stipulated in the Human Fertilisation and Embryology Act 1990. Although his wife Diane argued that such treatment would have been consistent with his wishes to have children, she was not a disinterested party in the outcome of any decisions regarding the sperm samples. This was subject to a review and widespread consultation by Professor Sheila McLean.[42] In patients temporarily unconscious, gamete removal was only justified if the individual's fertility was likely to be affected and it was not consistent with their best interests to delay gamete removal until contemporaneous consent could be given, but rather to allow them to have the ability to choose whether or not to parent. There was, however, a clear lack of certainty as to whether—in the permanently unconscious—the best interests test would be applicable, and 'the only benefit which can accrue is one to a third party, namely the remaining partner (and possibly to any potential child).[43] A recent case regarding removal of sperm from a man who was unconscious and likely to die before any recovery of consciousness seems to suggest that a permanently incapacitated individual's best interests may on occasion lie with a third party benefit. Gamete removal was considered lawful on the basis that the individual and his wife had previously sought referral for fertility treatment and there had been a priori discussion of, and agreement for, posthumous use of his sperm.[44]

In light of the Bland judgment and the legal view that in cases of permanent unconsciousness there can only really be a negative application of the best interests test if an individual becomes unconscious with no prospect of recovery, it may be logical to make decisions regarding medical treatments by reference to parties whose interests may be bound up in such decisions—for example, the relatives. Despite the requirements of the Mental Capacity Act, many ICU professionals would be uncomfortable with any greater strengthening of third party views because, outwith some cases of severe neurological injury, the process of reaching decisions regarding poor prospects of recovery is a gradual one.

Many would rather be comfortable with the dissenting legal view expressed by Justice Stevens in the Nancy Cruzan case that her interests did not disappear with her loss of consciousness because she would have 'an interest in how she will be thought of after her death by those whose opinions mattered to her'.[45] This is akin to the Court of Appeal's view of Anthony Bland's best interests, where it was clearly established that Anthony had never considered such a situation and there could be no assessment of his wishes regarding his continuing existence in the permanent vegetative state. If this were the case, treatment withdrawal would be legally supported as consistent with a patient's interests to be remembered in a certain way, or to be treated in a manner consistent with their previous dignity. Both these are views that are already held by many healthcare professionals, who believe that their current actions are consistent with such patterns of behaviour and thinking. However, this is not a policy of the courts nor expressed in statute, which merely requires that we operate with reference to third party views in determining where a patient's best interests lie, but it is unclear what if any interests such patients may still retain.

Summary

All adults are presumed to be competent and for medical treatment there is a general requirement to obtain consent. In a critical care setting, the necessity for life-saving treatments and the presence of intercurrent medical conditions mean that it may be easier to rebut any presumption of competence on the part of the patient to refuse life-saving treatment, but this cannot be assumed. Actions taken regarding patients lacking capacity should only be in the best interests of the patient and limited to what is deemed necessary at the time.

Prior to the introduction of the Mental Capacity Act 2005, the standard was that judged by a responsible and competent body of fellow professionals. The Act has formalized best interests along with a clearer definition of the requirements for capacity that brings greater clarification for critical care staff. It is lawful to prevent an individual lacking capacity from leaving intensive care provided that treatment is given in good faith and is materially the same treatment as would be given to a person of sound mind with the same physical illness.

Problems remain in implementing the best interests test and the emphasis given to what the person's wishes are 'thought' to be in the absence of any clear prior knowledge. Although the MCA requires consultation with individuals close to the patient who may have an idea what these wishes are, unless they have been granted a lasting power of attorney to make decisions concerning life-saving treatment, these only inform and do not wholly determine medical decision making. Unlike in the USA, we do not have formal legal recognition of substituted judgements of an incapacitated person's wishes although we are arguably moving closer to such a position.

In difficult cases involving treatment administration and withdrawal, critical care professionals are in a better position to make robust, defensible decisions if they consult fellow professionals as well as the immediate next of kin and independent mental capacity advocate they are required to. Under such circumstances, an individual patient's 'best interests' may involve many factors other than the purely medical.

References

1. Dworkin, G. *The Theory and Practice of Autonomy*, Cambridge University Press, Cambridge, 1988.
2. *Re T (Adult: Refusal of Treatment)* [1992] 4 All ER 649.
3. Cooke, MW, Wilson S, Cox P, Roalfe A. Public understanding of medical terminology: non-English speakers may not receive optimal care. *J Accid Emerg Med* 2000, 17, 119–21.
4. Adults with Incapacity (Scotland) Act 2000.
5. *R v Brown* [1994] 1 AC 212.
6. *B v NHS Hospital Trust* [2002] 2 All ER 449.
7. *Murray v McMurchy* [1949] 2 DLR 442.
8. *Willamson v East London and City Health Authority* [1997] 41 BMLR 85.
9. Non Consensual Treatment in Mason JK, Laurie GT, *Law and Medical Ethics*, Oxford University Press, Oxford, 2006, p. 353.
10. *Norfolk and Norwich Healthcare* (NHS) Trust v W 34 BMLR 16.
11. *Re MB (Medical Treatment)* [1997] 2 FLR 426.
12. *Kings College NHS Foundation Trust v C and V* [2015] EWCOP 80.
13. *Re F (Mental Patient: Sterilisation)* [1990] 2 AC 1.
14. *Airedale NHS Trust v Bland* [1993] AC 789 (CA).
15. Re MB (Medical Treatment) 12 BMLR 64.
16. *Re A (Medical Treatment: Male Sterilisation)* [2000] 1 FCR 193.
17. *R v Doctor M* [2003] 1 FLR 667.
18. *Simms v Simms* [2003] 2 WLR 1465.
19. General Medical Council. Treatment and care towards the end of life: good practice in decision making. 20 May 2010. https://www.gmc-uk.org/ethical-guidance/ethical-guidance-for-doctors/treatment-and-care-towards-the-end-of-life (accessed 7 December 2019).

20. McLean, SAM. *Consent and the Law*, Department of Health, 1997.

21. Per Chief Justice Rehnguist cited in Gunther, G, Sullivan, KM, *Constitutional Law*, 13th edition, Foundation Press, Westbury, New York, 1997) at p. 605.

22. *R (Burke) v General Medical council and Others* [2005] EWCA Civ 1003.

23. *Aintree University Hospitals NHS Foundation Trust v* James [2013] UKSC 67.

24. *Salford Royal NHS Foundation Trust v Mrs P & Anor (Rev 1)* [2017] EWCOP 23.

25. Honeybul S, Gillett KM, Ho KM et al. Long-term survival with unfavourable outcome: a qualitative and ethical analysis. *Journal of Medical Ethics* 2014, **41**, 963–9.

26. *Re T (Adult: Refusal of Medical Treatment)* [1992] 4 All ER 649.

27. *G v E* [2010] EWCOP 2512.

28. *P (by his litigation friend the Official Solicitor) v Cheshire West and Chester Council and another, P and Q (by their litigation friend the Official Solicitor) v Surrey County Council* [2014] UKSC 19.

29. Baharlo B, Bryden D, Brett SJ. Deprivation of liberty and intensive care: an update post Ferreira. *Journal of the Intensive Care Society* 2018, **19(1)** 35–42.

30. Law Commission. Mental capacity and deprivation of liberty. Law Com No 372, 3 March 2017. https://www.lawcom.gov.uk/project/mental-capacity-and-deprivation-of-liberty (accessed 31 October 2018).

31. https://www.gov.uk/government/news/new-law-introduced-to-protect-vulnerable-people-in-care (accessed 7 December 2019).

32. *The Secretary of State for the Home Department v Skripal* [2018] EWCOP 6.

33. Re MB (Medical Treatment) 12 BMLR 64.

34. Ibid.

35. *Law Hospital NHS Trust v Lord Advocate* 1996 SCLR 491–519.

36. Re MB (Medical Treatment) 12 BMLR 64.

37. Fenwick, AJ. Applying best interests to persistent vegetative state: a principled distortion? *Journal of Medical Ethics* 1998, **24**, 86–92.

38. Mason JK, Laurie GT. The management of the persistent vegetative state. *British Isles Juridical Review* 1996, 263–83.

39. https://www.bma.org.uk/advice/employment/ethics/mental-capacity/clinically-assisted-nutrition-and-hydration (accessed 7 December 2019).

40. NHS Trust A v M and NHS Trust B v H 58 BMLR 87.

41. Sheffield Teaching Hospitals Foundation Trust Staff Update on the Mental Capacity Act, prepared by Ms S Charles, October 2018.

42. Per Chief Justice Rehnguist.

43. Ibid.

44. *Y v A Healthcare NHS Trust & Ors* [2018] EWCOP 18.

45. *Cruzan v Director, Missouri Dept of Health* [1990] 110 S Ct 2841 at pp. 2885–6.

6

Promoting the Best Possible Death

Futility in Terminally Ill Patients Who Lack Capacity

Christopher Newdick and Christopher Danbury

Introduction

If we only read the news media, we might think that doctors are unfairly cavalier when they withdraw intensive care from patients, entirely indifferent to their wishes. In one recent case, the judge commented 'on the absurd notion ... that [the patient, Charlie Gard] has been a prisoner of the National Health Service or that the National Health Service has the power to decide Charlie's fate,' as a result of which hospital staff were threatened with violence.[1] Actually, the challenge may be the opposite. Doctors naturally seek to prolong every life until there is clear reason why not.[2] This means that cardiopulmonary resuscitation (CPR) is attempted for patients, even for whom it is futile, without regard for the condition of the patient, or the wishes of the relatives, unless there is a form confirming 'Do Not Attempt Cardiopulmonary Resuscitation (DNACPR)'. The National Confidential Enquiry into Patient Outcome and Death (NCEPOD) found in 2012:

> CPR was originally developed to save the lives of younger people dying unexpectedly, mostly from primary cardiac disease (the phrase 'hearts too young to die' is often used). However, CPR has come to be seen as a procedure that should be used for patients as a therapy to restore cardiopulmonary function and prolong life, irrespective of the underlying cause of cardiac arrest ... The result is that patients may undergo futile attempts at CPR during their dying process. Improved knowledge, training, and do not attempt cardiopulmonary resuscitation (DNACPR) decision-making should improve patient care and prevent these futile and undignified procedures at the end of life. Patients for whom CPR cannot prolong life, but merely prolong the dying process should be identified early.[3]

When does prolonged intensive care in terminally ill and incapacitated patients become futile? This chapter considers the risks surrounding intensive care decisions in respect of terminally ill patients who lack capacity. Intensive care saves the lives of about 80% of the patients it admits, and the pain and discomfort it causes in these cases must surely be justified. But what about the 20% for whom intensive care is unsuccessful because the patient is dying? Intensivists might be forgiven for prolonging treatment, not in the patient's best interests, but as a self-serving, least worse option to minimize the risk of complaint. After all, premature withdrawal of care may result in conflict with relatives, disciplinary proceedings, and even a charge of murder.[4] As Lady Black said in *An NHS Trust v Y*, even in the absence of complaint against a doctor, 'there is a risk that the need to go to court might deflect clinicians and families from making true best interests decisions and might lead in some cases to inappropriate treatment continuing by default.'[5]

Prolonging intensive care without regard to the suffering it causes would be wrong. Intensive care carries unavoidable side effects. Sedation in intensive care is not like a long, refreshing sleep. Dr Sarah Wake describes the sensation of intensive care and the delirium and stress it caused her:

> Endless days and nights filled with strange broken sleep. A sea of fragmented menacing faces and shadows swimming through erratic beeps and bells. A large cackling face floating over me, constantly morphing and changing shape. The staring old lady in the bed opposite, her sallow skin disintegrating, eyeballs disappearing to reveal deep dark holes from which cockroaches crawled. Her weary face melting like wax into a big grey smudge. Deafening, haunting laughter filling every space. Blood seeping through holes and cracks in my skin, forming a puddle of red around me. Small insects scuttling up my arms and legs. My chest locked to the bed with wires and straps, as a plastic mask repeatedly smothered me. A strangling sensation around my neck. A warm metallic taste. An invisible force pinning my body down as a dark curtain was drawn closed.[6]

And, David Aaronovitch, the *Times* columnist describes recovering from intensive care:

> I woke up to find that I was no longer mad. It was 2pm, my two brothers were sitting on either side of my hospital bed, my wife between them, the sun was slanting in through the window behind me and the horror that had dominated my life for nearly a week had evaporated. But I will never forget those days and nights of terror and delusion, and will never think about madness in the same way again.[7]

Especially in respect of those who are dying, when does the harm of intensive care cease to be justified by the benefit? At one end of the spectrum, some will die very quickly despite the care administered to them and the question of harmful intensive care is less likely to arise. At the other, a small minority may live on the intensive care ward for months during the process of dying. Although their passage toward death may be postponed, the trajectory is certain. Available statistics do not permit accurate estimates of the numbers of patients who die in intensive care after a prolonged stay. Among this group, how long should their suffering continue? Dying patients will often have limited capacity to articulate thoughts other than at a basic level of communication. How should we approach decision making in these cases? We discuss the systemic pressures that suggest that the number of patients in these circumstances is likely to be rising, and the challenges this presents.

Judging capacity to benefit—when does intensive care become 'futile'?

Who can benefit from intensive care? Who decides whether to admit or whether further treatment will be 'futile'? 'Futility is a subjective and nebulous concept which, except in the strictest physiological sense, incorporates value judgements ... '[8] At its most simple, futility in its 'strictest *physiological*' sense means that the treatment will not work and will provide the patient with no therapeutic benefit. There are numerous examples of physiological futility. These include the administration of an antibiotic to treat an infection that is resistant to that antibiotic; cardiopulmonary resuscitation in a patient who has an unwitnessed, non-shockable cardiac arrest; tachyphylaxis—a common example changing the rate of a noradrenaline infusion—given to raise blood pressure but which does not achieve its intended effect. This concept of futility was discussed in Tony Bland's case. As Sir Thomas Bingham MR said in the Court of Appeal:

> It is relevant to consider the objects of medical care. I think traditionally they have been (1) to prevent the occurrence of illness, injury or deformity (which for convenience I shall together call 'illness'), (2) to cure illness when it does occur, (3) where illness cannot be cured, to prevent or retard deterioration of the patient's condition and (4) to relieve pain and suffering in body and mind. I doubt if it has ever been an object of medical care merely to prolong the life of an insensate patient with no hope of recovery where nothing can be done to promote any of these objects.[9]

Lord Goff thought much the same in the House of Lords. He said: '... I cannot see that the medical treatment is appropriate or requisite simply to prolong a patient's life when such treatment has no therapeutic purpose of any kind, as where it is futile because the patient is unconscious and there is no prospect of any improvement in his condition.'[10] In *Bland,* the patient was in a persistent vegetative state (PVS) and treatment could offer him no clinical benefit. Charlie Gard's case is a slightly different example. The patient was a baby of eight months suffering a terminal, congenital condition. Francis J said of further treatment:

> It is the view of all those who have treated and been consulted in relation to Charlie in this country and also in Barcelona that such treatment would be futile, by which I mean would be of no effect but may well cause pain, suffering and distress to Charlie ... Accordingly, the entire highly experienced UK team, all those who provided second opinions and the consultant instructed by the parents in these proceedings share a common view that further treatment would be futile. For the avoidance of any doubt, the word 'futile' in this context means pointless or of no effective benefit.[11]

Many would agree that prolonging intensive care for PVS patients in is pointless.[12] But what about patients in a minimally conscious state (MCS) for whom treatment may be effective to prolong the patient's life, but (to put it another way) can only to extend the process of dying? This involves a different, nonclinical, test of futility. Say the patient is in MCS and dependent on treatment available in intensive care, but nowhere else. If the patient leaves the intensive care unit (ICU), they will die; if they remain, they may live for a prolonged and possibly indefinite period. Patients may be clinically stable on an ICU for years (despite the adverse psychological impact discussed above). How should we approach the many cases in this category? In truth, doctors cannot always be certain that a treatment will not work. More helpful is a *probabilistic* test of futility that discusses the likelihood of benefit arising from treatment. Treatment may not be considered futile when there is a low probability that it might succeed. This approach is common among intensive care doctors and reflects the scientific evidence on which their practice is based. But it raises complex questions that have no absolute answers: for example, is treatment futile if it has only a 5% likelihood of providing clinical benefit, or 1%, or 0.1%? And, of course, we may still argue whether an analysis of aggregates assists decision making about an individual patient. Knowing that 1 in 1,000 patients are likely to survive a particular illness with a particular treatment does not help me identify the individual who will survive. Should the 999 patients, who will die, be treated to the point of physiological futility to allow the one to survive? Or should the one patient not be treated in order to prevent the suffering of the 999, who are destined to die?

Intensive care physicians are uncomfortable treating to the point of physiological futility simply to prolong the process of dying. Their experience tells them earlier in the disease process that the patient will die, and they are distressed by prolonging treatment beyond that point. Moral distress occurs when the clinician believes that they know the right thing to do but constraints make it difficult or impossible to pursue the desired course. As Henrich et al. concluded, 'In response to moral distress, health care providers experience negative emotional consequences, patient care is perceived to be negatively affected, and nurses and other health care professionals are prone to consider quitting working in the intensive care unit.'[13] The point is illuminated in *An NHS Trust v DJ* (which proceeded to appeal as *Aintree NHS Hospital Trust v James*), where all ten doctors responsible for the patient's care believed further treatment to be futile. However, Peter Jackson J (as he was then), held that the patient had limited consciousness and enjoyed the company of his family and that, although he was dying, 'recovery does not mean a return to full health, but the resumption of a quality of life that DJ would regard as worthwhile.'[14] This contrasts the clinical view of the doctors with the non-clinical views of the family.

To add to the value judgments that surround well-understood clinical evidence, we must also acknowledge that doctors can get end of life decisions wrong. The Ethicus study[15] looked at end of life practices in intensive care across Europe. Of the 2,992 patients who had life-sustaining treatment withheld or withdrawn, 190 (6.4%) survived to be discharged from hospital. Of course this is a heterogenous group of countries, so the precise figure may be different in the UK. We do not know about the condition of these patients—for example, whether the patients go home to die, or need continual assistance at home, or do make a good recovery. Nevertheless, the fact remains that a number of patients on an ICU, who have had life-sustaining treatment withdrawn or withheld, have survived to discharge.

The challenge of making judgments in these cases is complicated by another consideration. How should we understand the factors that influence human decision making? We now accept that decision making is affected by the manner in which questions are framed. Framing is an example of a cognitive bias and was explored by Kahneman and Tversky. For example, in their 1981 experiment,[16] participants were asked to choose between two treatments for 600 people affected by a deadly disease. Participants were first asked to choose between Programs A and B:

If Program A is adopted, then 200 people will be saved (72% chose this option).

If Program B is adopted, there is a 1/3 probability that 600 people will be saved and a 2/3 probability that no people will be saved (28% chose this option).

The same participants were then asked to choose between Programs C and D:

If Program C is adopted, then 400 people will die (22% chose this option).

If Program D is adopted, there is a 1/3 probability that 600 people will be saved and a 2/3 probability that no people will be saved (78% chose this option).

Analysis shows that Programs A and C are the same. Similarly, Programs B and D are the same. Yet the participants were influenced by the ways in which the questions were presented. We are influenced by how problems are framed, patients and clinicians alike. This experiment and others led to the development of Prospect Theory,[17] which states that we make decisions based on the potential value of losses and gains rather than the final outcome. We are much more sensitive to avoid potential losses than equivalent gain. The evaluation of these losses and gains is influenced by consistent 'cognitive biases' and heuristics. Since then, our understanding of how people make decisions has continued to develop, with the discovery of increasing numbers of cognitive biases. One of the most important is called the 'Backfire effect'. When disagreement occurs, the Backfire effect[18] will tend to exacerbate the differences between clinicians and family. As conversations continue, so the relative positions may harden and become more polarized.

Inevitably, therefore, people will approach decisions about futility in different ways. The clinician is likely to approach it in an objective, analytical manner, looking at the experience of aggregates of patients and the likelihood of a gain for the patient in terms of symptom control and reduced suffering. By contrast, the family approach is likely to be more subjective and personal, thinking especially of the loss of their family member. In the uncertainty of intensive care, the subsequent decisions made by both the clinicians and the family may both be entirely reasonable yet diametrically opposed. These, therefore, are the considerations that lead cases to the courts.

Best interests—developments in case law

How has the law responded to the challenges presented by these judgments and uncertainties? The development of the best interests test can be described in three stages, although, as we shall see, the cases have not evolved in a consistent direction and there have been advances and retreats along the way.

Doctor's discretion

The first stage of development may be described as 'doctor knows best' under the 'Bolam' principle. As Lord Keith said in *Airedale NHS Trust v Bland*,[19] in a PVS case, no doctor is bound to treat a patient where no benefit would be conferred by doing so.

> Existence in a vegetative state with no prospects of recovery is by that opinion regarded as not being a benefit, and that, if not unarguably correct, at least forms a proper basis for the decision to discontinue treatment and care: see *Bolam v Friern Hospital Management Committee* [1957] 1 WLR 582.

Many would accept this statement in connection with patients in PVS, but the problem is that it does not stop with PVS. By making *Bolam* the reference point, it also embraces the range of different approaches reasonable doctors may take to treatment generally that have nothing to do with medicine or clinical benefit. For example, we know that religious convictions may influence the decisions made by intensive care doctors. A survey found that 'Catholic, Protestant and Moslem physicians had higher rates of withdrawal [of intensive care treatment] (53%, 49% and 37% respectively) rather than Jewish (19%) and Greek Orthodox (22%) ... Greater religiosity correlates with more prolonged care and reluctance to withdraw life-sustaining therapy.'[20] Doctors' 'non-clinical' views may be shaped by factors that have nothing to do with the patient's condition.[21] How is this relevant to intensive care decision making? In *Bland*, Lord Browne-Wilkinson acknowledged that:

> Different doctors may take different views both on strictly medical issues and the broader ethical issues which the question raises ... The doctor's answer may well be influenced by his own attitude to the sanctity of human life. In cases where there is no strictly medical point in continuing care, if a doctor holds the view that the patient is entitled to stay alive, whatever the quality of such life, he can quite reasonably reach the view that the continuation of intrusive care, being the only way of preserving such life, is in the patient's best interests. But, in the same circumstances another doctor who sees no merit in perpetuating a life of which the patient is unaware can equally reasonably reach the view that the continuation of

> treatment is not for the patient's benefit.... the court's only concern will be to be satisfied that the doctor's decision to discontinue is in accordance with a respectable body of medical opinion and that it is responsible.[22]

Although the relevance of personal and religious convictions has never been explained by the courts, support was given to this Bolam approach by the Court of Appeal in *Burke*. The Court of Appeal rejected the notion that patients have a right to insist on care the doctor considers inappropriate. It said:

> Autonomy and the right of self-determination do not entitle the patient to insist on receiving a particular medical treatment regardless of the nature of the treatment. Insofar as a doctor has a legal obligation to provide treatment this cannot be founded simply upon the fact that the patient demands it. The source of the duty lies elsewhere.[23]

Instead, the court endorsed a series of connected propositions: (1) doctors, exercising their professional clinical judgment decide what treatment options are clinically appropriate. (2) Doctors then offer this range of treatment options to the patient, explaining the risks, benefits, side effects, etc. involved in each. (3) The patient then decides which course of action to take, or to refuse them all. (4) If the patient consents to one of the treatment options offered, the doctor will proceed to provide it. (5):

> If, however, he refuses all of the treatment options offered to him and instead informs the doctor that he wants a form of treatment which the doctor has not offered him, the doctor will, no doubt, discuss that form of treatment with him (assuming that it is a form of treatment known to him) but if the doctor concludes that this treatment is not clinically indicated he is not required (i.e. he is under no legal obligation) to provide it to the patient although he should offer to arrange a second opinion.[24]

This gives doctors considerable discretion in deciding when the point of futility has been reached in intensive care. It means that some intensive care patients have life-sustaining treatment withdrawn when doctors are sure that no prospects of survival, even though this results in the patient losing a period of time, albeit unquantifiable, at the end of their lives. In Wales, for example, in *Abertawe Bro Morgannwg University LHB v RY and CP*, an application to withdraw treatment was made some six months before the time when the doctors assessed the patient would probably die. Given that population statistics may not be good predictors of the prospects of individual patients, is six additional months of life in such a patient with terminal illness futile—always, only sometimes, never?

We can at least say this: when agreement exists between clinicians and family about a patient's best interests, the court's involvement is not required. As Lady Black said in the Supreme Court:

> ... I do not consider that it has been established that the common law or the ECHR, in combination or separately, give rise to the mandatory requirement ... to involve the court to decide upon the best interests of every patient with a prolonged disorder of consciousness before clinically assisted nutrition and hydration (CANH) can be withdrawn.[25]

Court's discretion

What happens, then, when agreement between doctors and relatives cannot be achieved? Should the courts fall back on the Bolam principle? This approach has always attracted judicial critics. For example, Hoffmann LJ (as he was then) said in the Court of Appeal in *Bland*, disagreeing with the latitude proposed subsequently (above) in the House of Lords:

> The medical profession can tell the court about the patient's condition and prognosis and about the probable consequences of giving or not giving certain kinds of treatment or care, including the provision of artificial feeding. But whether in those circumstances it would be lawful to provide or withhold the treatment or care is a matter for the law and must be decided with regard to the general moral considerations of which I have spoken. As to these matters, the medical profession will no doubt have views which are entitled to great respect, but I would expect medical ethics to be formed by the law rather than the reverse ... This is a purely legal (or moral) decision which does not require any medical expertise and is therefore appropriately made by the court.[26]

The balance of power lies with the *court* to determine the patient's best interests. As Lady Black said in 2018 in *Re Y*:

> If, at the end of the medical process, it is apparent that the way forward is finely balanced, or there is a difference of medical opinion, or a lack of agreement to a proposed course of action from those with an interest in the patient's welfare, a court application can and should be made.[27]

Courts may disagree with the opinions expressed by doctors. For example, in a case involving a terminally ill baby whose life was coming to an end, doctors said that further treatment would be distressing to the baby, but the High Court said: '… it is positively in his best interests to continue with continuous pressure ventilation and with the nursing and medical care that properly go with it, including suctioning and deep suctioning when required, replacement of the tube as necessary, and chest and lung physiotherapy to clear his secretions.'[28]

Here, the court arbitrates between reasonable differences of clinical opinion to determine best interests. The position is explained in section 4(6) of the Mental Capacity Act 2005 that best interests require consideration of (among other things) '(a) the person's past and present wishes and feelings … , (b) the beliefs and wishes that would be likely to influence his decision if he had capacity, and (c) the other factors that he would be likely to consider if he were able to.' As Lady Hale said in the *James* case (discussed below), the advantage of this test is that it focuses on attention:

> upon the patient as an individual, rather than the conduct of the doctor, and [takes] all the circumstances, both medical and non-medical, into account. [And] that test should also contain 'a strong element of 'substituted judgment' (para 3.25), taking into account both the past and present wishes and feelings of [the patient …]'[29]

Clearly, so far as they are known, best interests should attend first to the patient's own beliefs, wishes, and feelings, rather than doctors' probabilistic analysis of best interests based on the clinical evidence of aggregates of patients.

Crucially, however, the court's arbitration is between reasonable differences of *clinical* opinions within the Bolam test.[30] What if no such difference of opinion exists because there is a *unanimous* clinical view that active treatment is not in a patient's best interests? Can such a view be challenged on non-clinical grounds? In *An NHS Trust v L, FL and TL*, the patient had suffered a series of heart attacks and was in low MCS. His relatives said that he would want everything done to preserve his life, even in his diminished condition. But there was 'unanimous… medical evidence that such treatment is not in Mr L's best interests … [and] it is unlikely any clinician would make a different decision.'[31] Responding to the unanimity of clinical view, Moylan J explained a well-established limitation to the exercise of the court's 'best interests' discretion. Confirming the principle in *Burke,* that available treatment options are for doctors to determine, he said:

> medical professionals cannot be required to provide treatment contrary to their professional judgement. It would clearly be inappropriate for the court to exercise its powers under the Mental Capacity Act in such a way as, to ... directly or indirectly require a doctor to treat a patient in a way that was contrary to the doctor's professional judgement and duty to the patient ... The Mental Capacity Act requires the court to exercise its independent judgement and to determine any application by reference to all the relevant circumstances. However, ... one of the circumstances needs to be a choice of treatment options. If there are no treatment options, then the court has no effective choice to make.[32]

True, in extreme cases, the court may disagree with the unanimous view of the doctors, but it may not order a doctor to provide treatment contrary to their clinical judgment. Before any order can be made, 'the parties must specifically address in the evidence what treatment options are available. Those options must be treatments which are available. They must be treatments which would not require medical professionals to act in a way which was contrary to their professional clinical judgement.'[33] Starkly put: 'If there is no-one available to undertake the necessary operation the question of whether or not it would be in the patient's best interests for that to happen is wholly academic and [further litigation] should be called to a halt here and now.'[34] Thus, the best interests test arises for consideration only after the treatment is considered appropriate. (Below, we consider use of this principle in connection with the availability of finite NHS resources.)

Patient's best interests—objective or subjective?

Understood in the manner described above, should the best interests test be an objective test according to the standards of a reasonable patient, or should it follow the patient's own views and feelings, even if they involve care that doctors find difficult to administer because of the suffering it causes? This question arose again in the case of DJ (discussed above) when it was taken to the Court of Appeal and then to the Supreme Court as *Aintree NHS Foundation Trust Hospital v James*. David James was 68 and was an intensive care patient. He had been on the unit for seven months and was dying. Although he was incompetent to make decisions about his life and death, his level of consciousness permitted him to communicate by smiling his pleasure at seeing his relatives. Lady Hale said of his condition, that he had suffered:

a stroke, which left him with right-sided weakness and contracture of his legs, and a cardiac arrest which required six minutes of advanced cardio-pulmonary resuscitation (CPR) to save him. He had recurring infections, leading to septic shock and multiple organ failure ... He had suffered from contractures, similar to very severe cramps, causing grimacing, raised pulse, breathing and blood pressure, indicating distress and pain. He had suffered a stroke, with severe neurological damage. He was completely dependent on artificial ventilation and required regular tube suction. His kidney function was extremely fragile, with a maximum function of 20% or so, although he had not so far required renal therapy. It was almost inevitable that he would face further infections leading to lowered blood pressure and the prospect of further multi-organ failure. Daily care tasks could cause discomfort, pain and suffering.[35]

As we noted above, all the doctors responsible for Mr James's care thought he had reached the end of his life and further attempts at resuscitation were not in his best interests (although the issue of outright refusal to treat was not advanced). Mr James had said to a member of the clinical staff that he would prefer to die if he could no longer play the guitar and the doctors were concerned that the burdens of continued resuscitation would be disproportionate to their benefits. They discussed with the relatives the possibility of withholding resuscitation when Mr James next entered a state of crisis and of administering palliative care only. The family challenged this view, perhaps hoping for a miracle.[36] In the trial court, the evidence of the conversation about wishing to die if he could not play music was simply dismissed— although there was no suggestion that this statement was not made. The narrative of the patient's wishes was taken from the family that the patient would not wish active treatment to be discontinued and the judge agreed.

On appeal, disagreeing with the trial judge, the Court of Appeal considered that, although the patient's life could be extended by further resuscitation, the personal costs of doing so would be disproportionate in terms of its burdens. We might call this the 'objective' test of futility. What would Mr James wish for himself, thinking as a reasonable patient? Given the inevitable course of the illness and the painful and distressing measures needed to further prolong it when the next crisis occurred, Ward LJ said:

one is driven to conclude that his wish to survive was unattainable ... In the overall assessment, therefore, of where best interests lie, I respect his wishes but in my judgment they must give way to what is in his medical best interests ... Viewed objectively, [his] life would become quite intolerable were he to suffer crisis leading to a further setback in his health ... the risks and burdens of trying to keep him alive would be disproportionate to the diminishing opportunities for him to take pleasure from his family. Thus, there was no longer the need to try, try and try again to restore him to the state he was bravely seeking to achieve.[37]

Arden LJ put the matter as follows:

Acting with humanity, and with respect for DJ's autonomy, I consider in the light of DJ's medical condition, his wishes would be unlikely to be to have the treatment of the kind in issue here, and that *a reasonable individual in the light of current scientific knowledge would reject it.*[38]

This version of the 'best interests' test adopts Sir Thomas Bingham's approach in *Bland* of an 'objective assessment of Mr Bland's best interests *viewed through his eyes.*'[39] The Court of Appeal said that Mr James, acting as a reasonable person, would not have wished to endure the pain and distress of further resuscitative treatment. This test is *objective* but incorporates a duty to pay particular attention to the patient's personal wishes.

However, the Supreme Court rejected this view. With the agreement of the other members of the Court, Lady Hale said that best interests referred to welfare 'in the widest sense, not just medical but social and psychological ... great weight [had] to be given to Mr James's family life which was of the closest and most meaningful kind.'[39] Her Ladyship agreed with Peter Jackson J in the High Court that it was too soon to say that a line had been crossed. Thus, although there may be no prospect of recovery, a limited level of improvement may still be worthwhile to the patient. Accordingly, she rejected the notion that the court's assessment of the patient's wishes and feelings was objective. Doctors 'must try and put themselves in the place of the *individual patient* and ask what his attitude to the treatment is or would be likely to be ... The purpose of the best interests test is to consider matters from the patient's point of view.'[40]

Equally, the objective/subjective distinction is not black and white. Consider the case of a terminally ill patient for whom further treatment 'serves no therapeutic purpose of any kind' (as the Court of Appeal found in *Aintree*). What *non-therapeutic* purposes can reasonably serve the patient's best interests to justify prolonging intensive care treatment? Is it simply for the patient, or their relatives to decide? There must be a limit because, as Lady Hale herself said in *Aintree*, agreeing with *Burke*: 'A patient cannot order a doctor to give a particular form of treatment ... We cannot always have what we want.'[41] And in a recent obstetrics case, Her Ladyship said the patient: 'cannot force her doctor to offer treatment which he or she considers futile or inappropriate.

But she is at least entitled to the information which will enable her to take a proper part in that decision.'[42] Recall too *An NHS Trust v L, FL and* TL: 'medical professionals cannot be required to provide treatment contrary to their professional judgement'.

What if a terminally ill intensive care patient has left instructions for their life to be extended on a ventilator irrespective of their suffering so they can see their daughter marry? Or a relative's request for cardiopulmonary resuscitation (CPR) likely to fracture fragile ribs and rupture internal organs? Perhaps it is helpful to contrast the Court of Appeal's concern for David James's personal *suffering* under a (modified) best interests test, with Lady Hale's emphasis upon non-therapeutic and subjective, personal *feelings*. This may tend towards an extension of treatment, but even Lady Hale in *Aintree* agreed that further exposure to the brutality of cardiopulmonary resuscitation would probably not have been in his best interests[43]—and indeed, no doctor may have been willing to attempt it in any event. Thus, some forms of treatment can be refused but, provided they have clinical support, others (perhaps less aggressive) may be considered, even if they may serve only to prolong the process of dying.

Relatives as a proxy for best interests

How can relatives assist in these cases? Section 4(7) of the Mental Capacity Act 2005 requires account to be taken, if practicable, of people named as someone to be consulted and anyone engaged in caring for the person or interested in their welfare. Clearly doctors should do their best to seek assistance from relatives who know and can speak about the patient's wishes.[44] Equally, relatives have no legal authority in law to consent, or refuse consent, to treatment. Doctors should be careful, therefore, to listen carefully to the views of relatives, but always within the framework of what is clinically appropriate and in the patient's best interests (and to proceed to judicial resolution when agreement cannot be achieved). For example, in *Aintree*, Mr James was no longer competent to make an informed decision about matters of life and death. Instead, his relatives represented him. Once the court believed it was hearing the authentic story of the patient's character and disposition, the next step of adhering to the patient's subjective wishes seems natural. The matter moves away from the best interests test toward a modified form of the patient's own (proxy) consent based on substituted judgment. A number of other cases have considered the best interests of the incapacitated patient on an ICU and deferred to the evidence of relatives. For example, in *St George's Healthcare NHS Trust v P and Q*, the court heard that a Muslim patient:

> strongly believed that life was sacred given by God and could only be taken away by God . . . that suffering was a component of predestination and someone else should not play an assisting role in shortening life merely because of the subjective quality of that life. It [was] against the tenet of his faith to do anything to shorten a life.[45]

Although he was in MCS and suffering end-stage renal failure, the court ordered the continuation of renal replacement therapy to reflect his wishes.

Similarly, in *Abertawe Bro Morgannwg University LHB v RY and CP*, the patient was in MCS and the question arose as to the clinical merits of a tracheostomy with deep-suctioning, which could cause serious pain and discomfort. The patient's daughter gave evidence that her father 'would want everything done' and that his Christian view would be that 'any life is better than none'.[46] Clinical evidence was submitted on the other side that generic statements of this nature cannot anticipate the extent of suffering intensive care may cause. Nevertheless, Hayden J considered that, although the procedure would be burdensome, it would not be 'overly burdensome' if it were required infrequently.[47] Clearly, each case presents a different matrix of facts and it is often difficult to generalize from one patient to another.

Nevertheless, the court retains a crucial role. For example, what if there is doubt whether the relatives have accurately expressed the patient's wishes, or a court believes the suffering and indignity to be expected from further treatment is disproportionate to any clinical benefit to be achieved? For example, in *Abertawe Bro Morgannwg University LHB*, the judge also said that, if the patient's condition deteriorated and deep suction became necessary on a daily basis, prolonged treatment of this nature would not be in the patient's best interests, and the hospital was invited to return to the court with an alternative treatment plan. This sheds light on Lady Hale's statement that 'we cannot always have what we want'. And in *An NHS Trust v A*, the relatives' strong religious view was for intensive care to continue. Yet the doctors considered it futile and reported that the patient was 'demonstrating a consistent purposeful effort in detaching or removing medical devices and resisting medical interventions' perhaps reflecting his wish to be free from further treatment. Balancing the arguments, the court said:

> . . . the views, if one can interpret them, of what the patient might be and the views of the family are highly material factors. At the end of the day they are not however

the governing factors when considering best interests ... in the patient's best interests the treatment ... should be withdrawn.[48]

But note too that this case was decided in 2005, before the Mental Capacity Act came into force, and the balance of decision-making power has now shifted toward subjectivity. Equally, a similar conclusion was reached in *An NHS Trust v L, FL and TL* (discussed earlier) in 2012. Recall that in Mr James's case, he had said that he would not wish to live if he could no longer make music. This evidence was dismissed, although it was not questioned. Space does not permit consideration of the evidence from environmental psychology that our 'character' is dynamic or relational, rather than static, and adapts to the people and environment that surround us.[49] An approach that seeks a 'perfectionist' view of our autonomous wishes by looking to past behaviours may overlook a range of different responses from terminally ill patients at the end of their lives. Accounts given of patients' wishes from different parties may arise from the willingness of patients to confide different things to different people. Patients might wish to shield from relatives, for example, their own suffering, or their altruistic wish to save further distress at the bedside. (And here, too, our responses may be influenced by the framing effect and cognitive biases we discussed earlier) These difficult questions are only recently being addressed in intensive care.[50]

Impact of best interests on NHS resources

One view of futility we have not considered is *economic*—that is, to what extent can the interests of one patient be modified in order to take account of the interests of others? Traditional bioethics focuses on individual claimants. Litigation too focuses on the rights of litigants and struggles to accommodate parties whose interests are not before the court. We put them to one side, hoping that Parliament will respond instead. Note the view of Lord Brown-Wilkinson in Tony Bland's case who said ' ... it is not legitimate for a judge in reaching a view as to what is for the benefit of the one individual whose life is in issue to take into account the wider practical issues as to allocation of limited financial resources or the impact on third parties ...'[51]

How best to utilize the finite beds available in intensive care wards? Say life-saving treatment is both clinically appropriate and in a patient's best interests. Is it sufficient for a patient or their relatives to state their wishes to continue to receive care, irrespective of the potential impact upon other needy patients?

An argument is available that it should, from the Court of Appeal in *Burke.* It said:

> No ... difficulty arises, however, in the situation ... of the competent patient who, regardless of the pain, suffering or indignity of his condition, makes it plain that he wishes to be kept alive. No authority lends the slightest countenance to the suggestion that the duty on the doctors to take reasonable steps to keep the patient alive in such circumstances may not persist. Indeed, it seems to us that for a doctor deliberately to interrupt life-prolonging treatment in the face of a competent patient's expressed wish to be kept alive, with the intention of thereby terminating the patient's life, would leave the doctor with no answer to a charge of murder.[52]

However, this statement applies to cases in which the treatment is both available and in a patient's best interests. In such cases, doctors may not simply refuse to treat. But this reintroduces the question, discussed earlier, as to what is 'available' (or, in the extract above, what are the 'reasonable steps' doctors should take)? We have discussed how the best interests test arises only after a reasonable body of clinical opinion is available to support it. This principle may also arise in connection with issues of *resources*. As a general rule, courts will not allocate scarce resources among the many legitimate claims submitted to them. That task belongs to public authorities and the role of judicial review is a *procedural* one to ensure that it is undertaken reasonably and lawfully. Many judicial review cases seek access to, for example, orthopaedic treatment, cancer therapy, cardiac, neonatal and paediatric care, in vitro fertilization, and transgender surgery.[53] In the vast majority, the courts defer to the reasonable discretion of health authorities as to how to allocate their finite resources. How should we understand this approach when it is in a patient's best interests to receive treatment, but NHS resources are not available to support it? An analogous issue arose in *N v ACCG* involving a claim from parents for NHS resources to enable them to provide intimate care to their son (P) at home. This would have involved the clinical commissioning group (CCG) in considerable expenditure in terms of training, equipment, and clinical support (and would have exposed P to clinical risk). The CCG refused to support the request. Refusing the application that this was in his best interests, Lady Hale asked:

> How is the court's duty to decide what is in the best interests of P to be reconciled with the fact that the court only has power to take a decision that P himself could have taken? It has no greater power to oblige others to do what is best than P would

have himself. This must mean that, just like P, the court can only choose between the 'available options . . .[54]

The court had no power to order a public authority to commit its resources in the manner requested. The statutory foundation for that decision properly belonged to the CCG. Application of the best interests test was irrelevant provided the CCG's decision was recognized as lawful. As with the position in respect of the availability of *clinical* discretion to provide treatment, the best interests test was conditional on a prior determination as to the availability of NHS resources. Intensive care has yet to be confronted with a legal challenge on precisely these grounds and the full potential in *N v ACCG* has not been explored. However, section 4(2) of the 2005 Mental Capacity Act requires best interest decision makers to have regard to 'relevant circumstances', and fair and equal access to NHS resources are surely relevant in this sense. In extreme circumstances, this could permit what we have called 'reverse triage', in which the least sick patients may of necessity have to be removed from intensive care to make way for patients with still more urgent need.[55]

The pressures on resources are illuminated by a 2009 European Society of Intensive Care Medicine study into the differences in intensive care medicine beds across Europe, with the UK having 6.6 per 100,000 population (compared with France at 11 and Germany at 27).[56] Modelling[57] demonstrates how treating one extra long-term patient has a disproportionate effect on the availability of critical care beds for other patients, particularly in small ICUs. Thus, as societal expectations change, and more patients are admitted to ICUs for longer periods of time, there will inevitably be an impact on the finite resources available to clinicians. As the only way ICUs have to control patient inflow is to limit access to an ICU, this will result in extending waiting times for critical care that are likely to be detrimental to other patients. Waiting times will go up for high-risk elective patients, and patients who may have benefitted from earlier admission will stay longer on a general ward or face transfers to ICUs in other hospitals. These eventualities inevitably reduce the chance of survival and the rate and degree of recovery. The Intensive Care National Audit and Research Centre data currently suggests that the mean length of stay on UK ICUs is 4.8 days. The number of long-stay patients is difficult to determine, but their effect is being felt increasingly. This is demonstrated by the rise in numbers of patients whose admission to intensive care has been cancelled for lack of ICU beds from 2,648 in 2010/11 to 3,980 in 2017/18.[58] Clearly this raises profound issues of law, ethics, economics, and, indeed, politics, but our failure to grapple with it is likely have adverse consequences for needy patients who are unable to access intensive care.

Dispute resolution

One of the challenges of our adversarial system of litigation is that it may encourage the expression of binary differences of opinion about a patient's wishes and feelings that may be partial and incomplete. What alternative means are available to resolve disputes of this nature? We have seen from *Re Y* that, when there is agreement between clinicians and families about best interests, there is no need to go to court. However, we also know from the Ethicus study that around 70% of people who die on an ICU do so following a decision to withhold or withdraw life-sustaining treatment, and from the international Conflicus study[59] that up to 80% of withdrawal/withholding decisions result in some degree of disagreement (although consensus is likely to be achieved after further discussion). However, what should be done when no agreement can be reached? Commencing litigation is one option, but this is more likely to polarizes opinion, escalate the dispute, and add to the stress suffered by patients, their relatives, and clinicians. How can the disagreements be approached in a sensitive manner so as to reduce this risk?

In 2010, Lord Justice Jackson published his review of civil litigation,[60] including healthcare disputes (although he concentrated on clinical negligence and personal injury cases). He discussed alternative dispute resolution (ADR), saying:

> For cases which do not settle early through bilateral negotiation, the most important form of ADR ... is mediation. The reason for the emphasis upon mediation is twofold. First, properly conducted mediation enables many (but certainly not all) civil disputes to be resolved at less cost and greater satisfaction to the parties than litigation. Secondly, many disputing parties are not aware of the full benefits to be gained from mediation and may, therefore, dismiss this option too readily.[61]

Facilitative mediation is the form most commonly practised in the UK. Mediation is a strictly confidential process that occurs without prejudice so that the discussions between the parties cannot be used in any subsequent litigation. The mediator does not take a position, but allows a conversation to take place between the participants. Prior to the mediation, parties will usually provide a written position statement to allow the mediator to understand their argument. The mediation is normally scheduled for four or eight hours and takes place in a series of rooms. It will often start with a caucus, or joint meeting, followed by the mediator shuttling between different rooms. It is a difficult process with the mediator challenging the respective views of the parties. The mediator reframes the position and will often play 'devil's advocate' to attempt to get the participants to look again at their positions. The process takes time and usually involves strong emotions on both sides. Mediation has a place in resolving disagreements about serious medical treatments on an ICU. The courts recognized this with Francis J commenting in the Charlie Gard case. He said:

> ... it is my clear view that mediation should be attempted in all cases such as this one even if all that it does is achieve a greater understanding by the parties of each other's positions. Few users of the court system will be in a greater state of turmoil and grief than parents in the position that these parents have been in and anything which helps them to understand the process and the viewpoint of the other side, even if they profoundly disagree with it, would in my judgment be of benefit and I hope that some lessons can therefore be taken from this tragic case which it has been my duty to oversee.[62]

Overseas experience with these cases is compelling with a Canadian report concluding that 60–80% of this type of mediation settles and 90% of participants found the experience helpful, even if they did not settle.[63] Mediation and other forms of ADR will generally settle faster and at less cost than traditional litigation. Mediation does not preclude litigation and indeed can proceed as a parallel process. The without prejudice nature of mediation means that anything discussed in that forum cannot be used in court, but it is a useful way of assisting a settlement without requiring the involvement of a judge.

NHS Resolution started mediating clinical negligence disputes in 2017 following a successful pilot in 2013/14. Forty-nine cases were accepted into the pilot. Of these, 47 completed mediations were undertaken of which 61% of the cases settled on the day of the mediation and 20% shortly thereafter.[64] The results since then have been very encouraging with far more cases mediated than expected over the following 18 months.[65] NHS Resolution uses mediators from an approved panel. Similarly, there has been discussion with the Court of Protection about the possibility of incorporating a practice direction encouraging mediation in all cases, including those of serious medical treatment.[66] One of the authors of this book, Christopher Danbury, is a registered mediator and has experience of successfully mediating SMT cases similar to those concerning Alfie Evans and Charlie Gard. His experience is that the process is more likely to result in the preservation of relationships and less likely to have the destructive impact that often follows litigation.

Conclusion

We commenced this chapter by asking how to promote the best possible death in intensive care and have discussed the systemic risks that, we fear, may work against that objective. The risk, which is discussed in the 2012 NCEPOD report, is impossible to quantify, but a number of factors may be identified as relevant causes. First, issues of informed consent are often extremely difficult so that decisions have to be made on behalf of patients by others doing their best to represent the patient's own wishes. In particular, we noted the different perceptions of clinical and non-clinical viewpoints. Second, we have seen how the focus of authority has shifted from doctors to the courts and, most recently, to patients themselves, heavily influenced by their relatives, and we have noted the imprecise and subjective nature of concepts used to resolve disputes such as futility and best interests. Third, the law has yet to be confronted by the resource allocation challenges presented by these cases. Judgments are given with no clear evidence of the extent to which promoting the autonomy of single litigants may adversely affect the access to intensive care of others in the queue. Last, we have noted the way in which doctors are likely to react to the threat of complaint by prolonging intensive care and the advantages of resolving disagreement outside the court by mediation. Given the inexact nature of the legal principles surrounding this area, this is likely to be the most satisfactory way of weighing the delicate balance between the burdens and benefits of continuing or withdrawing treatment. These considerations tend toward the preservation of the lives of terminally ill patients in intensive care. However, we are concerned that they may also expose patients to suffering many would choose to avoid while, at the same time, compromising the admission of others who could otherwise benefit from treatment.

References

1. *Great Ormond Street Hospital v Gard* [2017] EWHC 1909 at [18] (Fam).
2. See, for example, the 'purple form' in the 'Do not attempt cardiopulmonary resuscitation forms' at https://www.resus.org.uk/respect/ (accessed 5 January 2020).
3. Findlay GP, Shotton H, Kelly K, et al. (2012). *Time to intervene?* National Confidential Enquiry into Patient Outcome and Death, London . http://www.ncepod.org.uk/2012report1/downloads/CAP_summary.pdf (accessed 27 November 2019).

4. See *R v Nigel Cox* (1993) 12 BMLR 38.

5. [2018] UKSC 46 at [121].

6. Wake S, Kitchiner D. (2013). Post-traumatic stress disorder after intensive care. *British Medical Journal*, **346**, f3232.

7. Aaronovitch D. (2011). My nightmare in hospital. *The Times*, 12 November. The extensive literature on post-intensive care syndrome cannot be considered here.

8. *Willie Causey, Joe Cloman and Bernice Cloman, Plaintiffs-Appellants v St. Francis Medical Center and Dr Herschel R Harter, Individually and as a Medical Corporation, Defendants-Appellees* No. 30, 732-CA Court Of Appeal Of Louisiana Second Circuit 719 So. 2d 1072; 1998 La. App. LEXIS 2477.

9. *Airedale NHS Trust v Bland* [1993] 1 All ER 821at 836.

10. Ibid. at 871.

11. *Great Ormond Street Hospital v Yates, Gard and Gard* [2017] EWHC 972 (Fam) at [49] and [90]. These findings were accepted by the Supreme Court in its judgment refusing leave to appeal: https://www.supremecourt.uk/news/permission-to-appeal-hearing-in-the-matter-of-charlie-gard.html (accessed 27 November 2019).

12. But disagreement still persists. See, for example, Keown J. (2000). Beyond Bland: a critique of the BMA guidance on withholding and withdrawing medical treatment, *Legal Studies*, **66**.

13. Henrich NJ, Dodek PM, Gladstone E, et al. (2017). Consequences of moral distress in the intensive care unit: a qualitative study. *American Journal of Critical Care*, **26(4)**, e48–57. https://doi.org/10.4037/ajcc2017786 (accessed 27 November 2019).

14. *An NHS Trust v DJ* [2012] EWHC 3524 (COP) at [84].

15. Sprung C, Cohen S, Sjokvist P, et al. (2003). End-of-life practices in European intensive care units: the Ethicus study. *Journal of the American Medical Association*, **290(6)**, 790–7. https://doi.org/10.1001/jama.290.6.790 (accessed 27 November 2019).

16. Tversky A, Kahneman D. (1981). The framing of decisions and the psychology of choice. Science, **211(4481)**, 453–8.

17. Kahneman D, Tversky A. (1979). Prospect theory: an analysis of decision under risk. *Econometrica*, **47(2)**, 263. https://doi.org/10.2307/1914185 (accessed 27 November 2019).

18. First described in Nyhan, B, Reifler J. (2010) When corrections fail: the persistence of political misperceptions. *Political Behavior*, **32(2)**, (1 June), 303–30. https://doi.org/10.1007/s11109-010-9112-2 (accessed 5 January 2020).

19. [1993] 1 All ER 582, 821.

20. Sprung C, Maia P, Bulow H, et al. (2007). The importance of religious affiliation and culture on end-of-life decisions in European intensive care units, *Intensive Care Medicine*, **33(10)**, 1732, 1737–8.

21. See Keown J. (1997). Restoring moral and intellectual shape to the law after *Bland*, *Law Quarterly Review*, **113**, 481.
22. *Airedale NHS Trust v Bland* [1993] 1 All ER 821, 882–883.
23. *Burke v General Medical Council* [2005] Lloyds Rep Med 403at [31].
24. Ibid. at [50].
25. *An NHS Trust & Ors v Y & Anor* (Rev 1) [2018] UKSC 46 (UKSC (2018) 30 July 2018) at [126].
26. Hoffmann LJ, 858. See also, *Frenchay Health Care NHS Trust v S* [1994] 2 All ER 403: ' … there should not be a belief that what the doctor says is the patient's *is* the patient's best interest' (Sir Thomas Bingham MR, 411) and *Law Hospital NHS Trust v The Lord Advocate* 39 BMLR 166 (1998); 4 Med L.Rep 300, '… it may be that, in the past … doctors exercised their own discretion in such cases, in accordance with medical ethics, where there was a body of informed and responsible medical opinion that to continue treatment would confer no benefit … But the question whether it would be lawful to cease to provide or to withhold treatment cannot be left to the doctors. This is a matter for the law, and it must be decided by the courts, so long as there is no declaration on the matter by Parliament' (171, Lord President Hope).
27. Ibid. at 125.
28. *An NHS Trust v MB* [2006] EWHC 507 at [90], Holman J. But see *Great Ormond Street Hospital v Gard* [2017] EWHC 1909 deciding further treatment was not in a child's best interests.
29. *Aintree University Hospitals NHS Foundation Trust v James* [2013] UKSC 76 at [24].
30. See the discussion in *Re S (Adult Patient: Sterilisation)* [2001] Fam 15.
31. [2012] EWHC 4313 (Fam) at [88]. Note the case was decided before *Aintree v James*.
32. Ibid. at [112]–[113]. See also, *Re J (A Minor)(Wardship: Medical Treatment)* [1991] Fam 33.
33. Ibid. at [116].
34. *AVS v A NHS Foundation Trust* [2011] EWCA Civ 7 at [39].
35. *Aintree University Hospitals NHS Foundation Trust v James* [2013] UKSC 76 at [2]–[3].
36. See *An NHS Trust v DJ* [2012] EWHC 3524 (COP) at [80] and *Aintree University Hospitals NHS Foundation Trust v James* [2013] EWCA 65 at [29] and [47].
37. *Aintree Hospital v James* [2013] EWCA Civ 65 at [47]–[49].
38. *Aintree Hospital v James* [2013] EWCA Civ 65, [63] emphasis added.
39. *Aintree University Hospital NHS Foundation Trust v David James* [2013] UKSC 67 at [39]–[40].
40. Ibid. at [39]–]45], emphasis added.

41. Ibid. at [14] and [45].

42. *Montgomery v Lanarkshire Health Board* [2015] UKSC 11 at [115].

43. *Aintree Hospital v James* [2013] UKSC 67 at [41–42].

44. *Winspear v City Hospitals Sunderland NHS FT* [2015] EWHC 3250 (QB).

45. [2015] EWCOP 42 at [38].

46. *Abertawe Bro Morgannwg University LHB v RY and CP* [2017] EWCOP 2 at [5]. The case demonstrates how the court may seek to understand patients' views through the voice of close relatives.

47. The phrase is used in the *Code of Practice to the Mental Capacity Act*, para 5.31. In fact, the patient died peacefully in hospital shortly after the judgment was handed down.

48. [2006] Lloyd's Rep Med 29, 59 and 99. See also, *Lincolnshire v N* [2014] EWCOP 16 for another case in which the MCS patient's actions were indicative of a wish to *refuse* treatment.

49. See, for example, Barker R. (1968). *Ecological psychology: concepts and methods for studying the environment of human behavior.* Stanford University Press. Exploring the question, see Hesse H. (1977). *Steppenwolf.* Penguin, London, inviting us to 'break through the illusion of unity of personality and perceive that the self is made up of a bundle of selves . . . ' (page 71).

50. See Birchley G. (2018). What God and the angels know of us? Character, autonomy, and best interests in minimally conscious state. *Medical Law Review*, 26, 392, arguing that this 'perfectionist' account may not truly represent patients' wishes. The court preferred the views of carers over relatives in *W v M* [2011] EWHC 2443.

51. *Airedale NHS Trust v Bland* [1993] 1 All ER 821, 879. See also, Lord Mustill at 893.

52. *Burke v General Medical Council* [2005] Lloyds Rep Med 403 at [34].

53. See generally, Newdick C. (2005). *Who should we treat? Rights, rationing and resources in the NHS.* Oxford University Press.

54. *N v ACCG* [2017] UKSC 22 at [35]. Similarly, see *Holmes-Moorhouse v Richmond upon Thames* [2009] UKHL 7, disapproving of judicial orders to provide council housing.

55. Newdick C, Danbury C. (2010). Reverse triage? Managing scarce resources in intensive care, in (eds) Danbury C, Newdick C, Lawson A. et al. *Law and ethics in intensive care* (1st edn), 191–211. Oxford University Press.

56. Rhodes A, Ferdinande P, Flaatten H, et al. (2012). The variability of critical care bed numbers in Europe. *Intensive Care Medicine*, 38(10), 1647–53. https://doi.org/10.1007/s00134-012-2627-8 (accessed 27 November 2019).

57. Shahani A, Ridley S, Nielsen M. (2008). Modelling patient flows as an aid to decision making for critical care capacities and organisation. *Anaesthesia*, 63(10),

1074–80. https://doi.org/10.1111/j.1365-2044.2008.05577.x (accessed 27 November 2019).

58. NHS England. Critical care bed capacity and urgent operations cancelled 2017-18 data. https://www.england.nhs.uk/statistics/statistical-work-areas/critical-care-capacity/critical-care-bed-capacity-and-urgent-operations-cancelled-2017-18-data (accessed 27 November 2019).

59. Azoulay E, Timsit J-F, Sprung CL, et al. (2009). Prevalence and factors of intensive care unit conflicts: the Conflicus study. *American Journal of Respiratory and Critical Care Medicine*, **180(9)**, 853–60.

60. Ministry of Justice (2010). *Review of civil litigation costs*. The Stationery Office, Norwich.

61. Ibid. Chapter 36, 1.2.

62. *Great Ormond Street Hospital v Gard* [2017] EWHC 1909 at [20]

63. Watts, L. (2013). Elder and guardianship mediation, in (eds) Arai M, Becker U, Lipp V. *Adult guardianship law for the 21st century*, 217–21. Nomos Verlagsgesellschaft mbH & Co. KG.

64. Centre for Effective Dispute Resolution (2017). Mediation in public healthcare—making a positive difference. https://www.cedr.com (accessed 27 December 2019).

65. NHS Resolution (2018). NHS Resolution presses ahead with mediation as litigation decreases but claims costs continue to rise. https://resolution.nhs.uk/nhs-resolution-presses-ahead-with-mediation-as-litigation-decreases-but-claims-costs-continue-to-rise (accessed 27 November 2019).

66. Personal communication.

7

Diagnosing Death

Dale Gardiner and Andrew McGee

Introduction

It was not always doctors who diagnosed death. Hippocratic tradition required that, as death approached or seemed to approach, doctors withdrew from patient care and gave way to the family and priests.[1] Two social forces, operating through the eighteenth and nineteenth centuries, led to the diagnosis of death becoming a duty of doctors and, by extension, other designated healthcare professionals.

A doctor's duty

The first social force emerged from medical interest in resuscitation, which had predominantly been a domain of midwifery. Primitive and ineffective by today's standards, the latter part of the eighteenth century saw doctors attempting resuscitation after cardiorespiratory arrest, particularly following drowning. Techniques ranged from rolling a patient over a barrel or side to side, providing heat and physical stimulation, or using ventilation bellows. Unfortunately, ventilation led to cases of such serious barotrauma that the technique fell into relative disregard through much of the nineteenth century.[2] It wasn't until the twentieth century that cardiopulmonary resuscitation (CPR), as we understand it today, became accepted as a medical core skill—or, as Peter Safar, one of the greats in resuscitation history would term it—'cardiopulmonary-cerebral resuscitation'.[3] Despite the stuttering start, the fire had been lit, and an expectation created that it was doctors who could resuscitate and save the near dead, perhaps even reverse death. Doctors were called more frequently when death approached, and it predictably fell increasingly upon doctors to declare that resuscitation was futile, and death had occurred.

The second social force concerned the long-held human fear of being buried alive. This fear reached new levels of public hysteria in the eighteenth century with myth and case reports abounding of people waking from apparent death, or coffins being opened with signs that the occupant had tried to escape their gruesome fate. Jacques Bénigne Winslow and Jean-Jacques Bruhier famously contended that putrefaction was the only sure sign of death[4]—a conclusion that may have been a reason for George Washington's alleged dying request: 'Have me decently buried, but do not let my body be put into a vault in less than three days after I am dead.'[5] As a way to ease public fear in Germany, 'waiting mortuaries' were constructed. The apparently dead had to be placed in stone and unrefrigerated buildings for a number of days (often three) before burial was allowed.[6]

In the mid-nineteenth century, the Academy of Sciences in Paris challenged this practice on the ground that, in 50 years of mortuary homes in Germany, nobody had yet recovered to life, but families still had to pay for the body to be received.[7] Putrefaction, one of the somatic criteria for death, was obviously proving a very safe diagnostic criterion but not a very timely one. The Academy of Sciences offered a reward to the physician who successfully made 'the diagnosis of death safe, prompt and easy'.

The prize was won by Eugène Bouchut in 1846 for his *Trâité des Signes de la Mort* [*Treatise on the signs of death*].[8] He made two compelling arguments that were accepted by the Academy. The first was that it should be doctors who diagnose death and they should be paid for doing so. This would aid public safety in preventing premature burial, and assist with death certification and coronial investigations. His second argument addressed the need for ease and timeliness. Bouchut advocated the use of the stethoscope, invented in 1819 by René Laennec, as a technological aid to diagnose death. When the heartbeat was absent for five minutes, a person could be diagnosed dead.

As the twentieth century commenced, it was doctors who were entrusted by society to diagnose death. While not codified as such, the new duties of doctors can be summarised as a prima facie duty to resuscitate and save those who can be saved and, for those who cannot be saved, to declare death in a safe and timely manner (see Box 7.1).

Box 7.1. A doctor's duty in diagnosing death

Resuscitate—save those you can

Declare death—diagnose the dead

1. *Safely*—no coming back to life after death declared
2. *Timely*—no unnecessary delay

A safe and timely diagnosis

The tension between safety and timeliness is not easy to navigate. Errors in diagnosis should never occur—yet to err is human and all diagnostic criteria have a sensitivity and specificity. Questions of timeliness are no less challenging. When can grieving start, the family leave the bedside, autopsies commence (very rapidly in warm autopsies), organs be recovered, and the body buried? Dying is a process that affects different functions and cells of the body at varying rates of decay. Into this process, doctors must step and decide at what moment there is permanence and death can be declared.

The birth of intensive care in the 1950s only made this job harder. A new type of patient was appearing. Unlike in all human history, brain arrest and circulatory arrest no longer had to coincide. On the intensive care unit (ICU), mechanically ventilated patients were identified who had demonstrably and permanently lost brain circulation and brain function, including the ability to breathe spontaneously, yet their hearts continued to beat. The French, again leading the way, termed this condition '*coma dépassé*—a state beyond coma.[9] Clinicians began asking whether these patients were already dead. For the first time, they had to decide whether *both* heart and brain functions had to cease before the patient could be said to have died, or whether it was sufficient if brain function and the ability to breathe had been lost.

On 5 August 1968, the ad hoc committee of the Harvard Medical School published its landmark paper, 'A definition of irreversible coma', which proposed that a permanently non-functioning brain represented the death of the individual.[10] The chair of the ad hoc committee, and the key driver behind this proposal, was Henry Beecher, the first endowed chair of anaesthesiology in the world and founder of the first ICU at Massachusetts General Hospital.[11] This link is no surprise. The burden of knowing what to do with these patients is felt most acutely by ICUs, their patients, families, and staff. Or, as Henry Beecher graphically put it, ' ... if beds are not cleared of corpses, cancer patients will be denied hospital admission.'[12] The need for a timely diagnosis of death was obviously a prime concern for him.

On the very same day that the ad hoc committee published its paper, the 22nd World Medical Assembly was meeting in Sydney, Australia. The Assembly had been working in parallel and apparently unaware of the ad hoc committee's work. Their announcement became 'The declaration of Sydney on human death.'[13] This declaration contained two important statements— a) that the determination of the time of death should remain the legal responsibility of doctors, and b) that there is a distinction between death at the cellular and tissue levels and the fate of a person.

Toward a unifying concept of human death

Neurological criteria for death gradually gained acceptance in most parts of the world with developed intensive care infrastructure, albeit the rate of acceptance varied from place to place. In the UK, the acceptance of neurological criteria occurred in 1976, in a statement from the Conference of Medical Royal Colleges and their Faculties where it was 'agreed that permanent functional death of the brain stem constitutes brain death.'[14] Very importantly in the UK, the Royal Colleges issued a memorandum in 1979 stating that '[w]hatever the mode of its production, brain death represents the stage at which a patient becomes truly dead.'[15] This was an early attempt to unite the concept of human death to the brain.

The latest 2008 UK Code of Practice develops this tradition:

> The definition of death should be regarded as the irreversible loss of the capacity for consciousness, combined with irreversible loss of the capacity to breathe ... The irreversible cessation of brain-stem function whether induced by intra-cranial events or the result of extra-cranial phenomena, such as hypoxia, will produce this clinical state and therefore irreversible cessation of the integrative function of the brain-stem equates with the death of the individual and allows the medical practitioner to diagnose death.[16]

In the USA, a different approach was taken. State legislation, based on the Uniform Determination of Death Act 1981 (UDDA), widely established neurological criteria as the basis for declaring death in statute, but in doing so created a duality in the diagnostic definition of death (which many countries have emulated):

An individual who has sustained either (1) irreversible cessation of circulatory and respiratory functions, or (2) irreversible cessation of all functions of the entire brain, the brain stem, is dead. A determination of death must be made in accordance with accepted medical standards.'[17]

Recently in North America there has been a revisiting of this duality and a renewed focus on the brain. In 2008, the US President's Council on Bioethics concluded that the fundamental vital work of a living organism is achieved through the organism's need-driven commerce with the surrounding world.[18] For a human being, this commerce is manifested by the drive to breathe, demonstrating the most basic way a human being can act upon the world, combined with consciousness, or the ability to be open to the world. The irreversible loss of these two functions, according to the President's Council, equates to human death.[19] This of course is remarkably similar to the UK position. While the Council did not extrapolate their conclusion to justify criteria for death following cardiorespiratory arrest, other North American authors have. Bernat et al. concluded that 'although stated separately, the two standards [in the UDDA] are essentially a single one based on brain functions'.[20] This is in keeping with Peter Safar's description of cardiopulmonary-cerebral resuscitation where the emphasis and goal of resuscitation are to save the brain.[21]

The history of practice development in the diagnosis of death reveals that alterations in the definition of death, and our ethical and legal understanding of such, are a response to technological advances that continue to challenge and refine our understanding of human death. A recent, Canadian-led endeavour, developed in collaboration with the World Health Organization (WHO), advanced a single operational definition of human death:

> Death occurs when there is permanent loss of capacity for consciousness and loss of all brainstem functions. This may result from permanent cessation of circulation or catastrophic brain injury. In the context of death determination, 'permanent' refers to loss of function that cannot resume spontaneously and will not be restored through intervention.[22]

This single definition of death could be termed 'permanent brain arrest'. The clinical characteristics of permanent brain arrest would therefore be the permanent loss of capacity for consciousness and loss of all brainstem functions (including the capacity to breathe), which might arise from primary brain injury or secondary to circulatory arrest.[23]

A way of conceptually understanding a unified concept of human death is given in Figure 7.1. This illustrates the use of three sets of criteria by doctors to diagnose death, depending on the clinical circumstances. All three sets of criteria point to the same definition of death—permanent brain arrest. In forensics or where death may have occurred many hours or days before, somatic criteria are used—the ancient, and externally obvious, signs of death —for example, rigor mortis, decapitation, and decomposition.[24] In hospital, where cardiorespiratory arrest has occurred and resuscitation has failed, or it has been decided that it will not be attempted, doctors follow the teaching of Eugène Bouchut and use a stethoscope to diagnose death—safe in the knowledge that, after five minutes of continuous mechanical asystole,

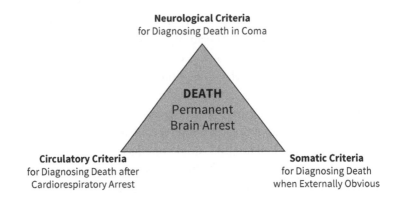

Figure 7.1

Adapted from *British Journal of Anaesthesia*, 108, Suppl 1, Gardiner D, Shemie S, Manara A, and Opdam H, International perspective on the diagnosis of death, i14-28, Copyright 2012, with permission from The Authors, published by Elsevier

autoresuscitation will not occur.[25] In rare circumstances, found only in intensive care environments where primary neurological injury has led to permanent brain arrest, neurological criteria for death can be applied.

The clinical characteristics of 'permanent brain arrest' are the permanent loss of capacity for consciousness and loss of all brainstem functions (including the capacity to breathe), which might arise from primary brain injury or secondary to circulatory arrest. The above discussion has outlined the current medical standards and some of the historical and ethical justification for those standards. While there is widespread consensus for these standards—in practice and in law—they are not without criticism from a small but vocal minority. The following section outlines the main arguments of criticism and offers possible brief defences.

Being dead

Dead already

While less prevalent in recent literature and discourse, there is an argument that the diagnosis of death using neurological criteria is too restrictive and too slow. This argument maintains that the loss of personhood, defined as loss of consciousness, is what counts.[26] Leaving aside the frequent misreporting in the media where a vegetative state is referred to as 'brain death', this would be the claim that those in vegetative states (or perhaps severe forms of Alzheimer's) lack conscious awareness and therefore can be regarded as having already died.

This argument has never gained great traction. First, in terms of achieving a safe diagnosis, misdiagnoses in vegetative and minimal conscious states are far too common, with errors in the order of more than one third.[27,28] Second, consciousness is, in medical circles at least, accepted as being manifested by two physiological components: awareness and arousal (wakefulness).[29] Arousal and wakefulness are brainstem-mediated functions. A patient in a vegetative state may lack awareness, even if correctly diagnosed and with no evidence of improvement over time, but will demonstrate signs of arousal because their brainstem is functioning. The emphasis given to the brainstem in neurological criteria for death is no accident and reflects the consensus that consciousness is more than just awareness.[30,31] Patients in vegetative states are conscious, even if only at a rudimentary level, and for this reason there seems no likelihood that the definition of death would ever be altered to include this cohort of patients. (This point has not been sufficiently appreciated by some philosophers who wrongly describe persistent vegetative states patients as unconscious.)

Not dead—philosophical objection

A more fundamental objection to the identification of neurological criteria with death—and so to the cogency of brain-based criteria for declaring death—is that, even if we assume that brainstem function and consciousness, including arousal, has permanently ceased, it is difficult to see why that should be the death of the human organism.[32,33,34,35] A brain-dead human organism continues to have many intact functions, including continuing heartbeat and circulation, digestion, and wound healing. Moreover, there have even been successful continuations of pregnancy resulting in live and healthy births. These objections have been the source of considerable debate.[36,37,38] We have insufficient space to discuss them here but one can distinguish between our being human beings and our being human organisms (as does the declaration of Sydney, see page X).[39] An early embryo is uncontroversially a human organism, but it is not yet a human being—at the very least not until the point where the possibility for twinning has passed and there has been some cell differentiation.

Similarly, ubiquitous thought experiments, which started in philosophical literature before being transferred over into the 'brain death' literature, have suggested that we do not need to accept the claim that we are *essentially* human organisms (even if we *are* essentially human beings), at least if that means that we could not imagine technological developments that might prompt us to revise our concepts. These technological developments are already occurring following the birth of intensive care (see page X). We can also avoid, altogether, the notorious thought experiments of brain transplants which, however persuasive, always seem to fall that little bit short owing to their hypothetical status. We can instead refer to several real, but unpleasant, cases involving animals, such as White's transplantation of a monkey head onto a different monkey torso, or Demikhov's creation of a hybrid dog achieved by joining half the torso with the tail and half of another dog's torso with the head.[40] There is, of course, no factual or empirical answer to the question of which of these monkeys or dogs is the original one, but our knowledge that the brain is responsible for our awareness and arousal—conditions for our mental life—strongly suggests that we should decide this issue by stipulation: the monkey or dog whose head is transplanted and continues to be conscious in the wide sense is the original dog, whose life continues adjoined to a different organism. If, as has been rumoured, the first ever human head transplant occurs, we might stipulate at that point that the human being goes with the head, and should from that point on be distinguished from the human organism (the rest of the body from which the head was transplanted).[41]

These points reveal another important truth: we have already started to embark on this very shift with the adoption of brain-centric definitions of death. When consciousness in the wide sense, which includes arousal, has ceased, we classify the human being as dead. Critics such as Shewmon and Miller and Truog may be right that the human organism remains alive but, because our society has started to shift *what counts* as a human being having died, it has started to distinguish between the human being and the human organism at the end of life, just as, for many years, it has made the same distinction at the beginning of life. Although we are more than our brains in the sense that we are nothing without our bodies, we are no more than our brains in the different sense that we can live with a different body, at least in principle. The monkey head and dog transplants have shown this to be so. The rest of the human organism—the torso with arms and legs and the rest of our circulatory system—is separable in principle because there is nothing incoherent about stipulating that, on a successful head transplant, the human being survives in the transplanted head, with a new torso. Note that we could stipulate the converse instead: we could stipulate that the human being dies because they have lost their torso. But there are better reasons for adopting the first stipulation than the second, including the puzzle of what we ought to say about to whom the conscious head belongs, if we do indeed stipulate the converse and say that the human being has died.

The fact that we sometimes need to make stipulations should not in any way be surprising. Science is full of examples where our concepts have changed over time. An example is the definition of acid. Acid used to be defined as the liquid that turns litmus paper red, but subsequently became defined differently, as proton donors.[42] Experiments such as Demikhov's and White's can prompt us likewise to change our definition of what it is to be a human being, and support the claim that human beings die when the brain dies. This is the route society has taken in accepting a brain-centric definition of death.

Even if a brain-centric definition is accepted, a worldwide question remains: which bit of the brain counts? The UDDA requires 'irreversible cessation of all functions of the entire brain, including the brain stem'[43] while the UK requires 'irreversible cessation of the integrative function of the brainstem'[44] and the proposed World Health Organization definition is 'permanent loss of capacity for consciousness and loss of all brainstem functions.'[45]

This apparent philosophical difference is less than it appears. From a clinical perspective, while it is possible to diagnose death in the UK in patients with isolated injuries to the brainstem, this is very rare.[46] Even in the USA, the actual recommendations for diagnosing death using neurological criteria are clinical bedside tests of the brainstem only and there is no requirement for ancillary investigations to demonstrate absent brain blood flow or absent, coordinated, electrical cortical function.[47] The effect is that individuals diagnosed dead in the UK and in the USA, by their respective neurological criteria, are almost always clinically indistinguishable. A recent case series from the USA made this point even clearer by observing how patients with isolated posterior fossa catastrophic lesions (potentially satisfying UK brainstem-based neurological criteria) all eventually developed loss of supra-tentorial blood flow over a few days, thereby satisfying both definitions fully.[48]

A different objection is the emphasis in the UDDA that to be dead there must be loss of 'all functions of the entire brain'. Yet not all patients who are diagnosed deceased in the USA using neurological criteria develop diabetes insipidus, which means their brain must still be secreting anti-diuretic hormone; therefore, the patient has not lost all functions of the brain.[49] There is a possible anatomical explanation. The posterior pituitary and, to a lesser degree, the anterior pituitary (indirect partial supply via short portal vessels), is supplied by the inferior hypophysial artery, which is extradural in origin.[50,51] Whatever the blood supply explanation, the objection is that, even by following the current US criteria, in some cases patients are being diagnosed deceased who do not satisfy the UDDA definition of death.[52,53]

The preoccupation with 'all' is hard to comprehend when it is not a requirement of the cardiorespiratory criteria of the UDDA, which is simply 'irreversible cessation of circulatory and respiratory functions'. The heart has hormonal
function—for example, the heart hormone atrial natriuretic peptide (ANP)—
not just its beating function. Ischaemia is one of the most potent stimuli for
ANP secretion and cardiac arrest is a potent cause of cardiac ischaemia.[54]
Yet has any doctor delayed diagnosing death after cardiac arrest in case there
may be persisting hormonal function of the heart? In diagnosing death after
cardiac arrest, therefore, certain functions are already being prioritised over
others. The UK and WHO's position would be that the brain should be no different. Only some functions of the brain need count to satisfy a definition of
permanent brain arrest, being permanent loss of capacity for consciousness
and loss of all brainstem functions (including the capacity to breathe). These
capacities and functions are anatomically located to the brainstem.

There may be residual *legal* problems in the USA given the statutory requirement in the UDDA that *all* functions of the *entire* brain must have ceased.
Challenges have been brought in the USA in which one court has expressed
strong doubts about medical guidelines that do not appear to comply with
this statutory requirement. Lawmakers in the USA might need to consider
amending its legislation to bring it more in line with the UK and WHO position and current death declaration practice both in the USA and around the
world, in order to avoid any ongoing legal problems and challenges.[55]

Not dead—medical objection

A separate controversy has arisen in the context of diagnosing death using
circulatory criteria where it is claimed that current criteria confuse a prognosis with a diagnosis.[56,57] This concerns the word 'irreversible' in the UDDA
and the more general putative conceptual requirement that death must be
irreversible in order to have occurred.[58,59,60,61,62,63] The relevant limb of the
UDDA requires the 'irreversible cessation of circulatory and respiratory functions', although there is an essential qualification in the definition that requires
that the 'determination of death must be made in accordance with accepted
medical standards'.[64] The combination of these two requirements makes the
UDDA ambiguous, because accepted medical standards allow death declaration on the basis of the *permanent* cessation of circulatory-respiratory function.[65] The ambiguity arises because, as a matter of law, it could be argued
that 'irreversible' in this context means *permanent*. The words 'permanent'
and 'irreversible' were used interchangeably in the report leading up to the

enactment of the UDDA[66] so, if the issue ever came to court, judges would be allowed to have access to these materials in deciding what the word 'irreversible' in the UDDA means. But the oscillation in the report between these two terms means that the report itself is ambiguous, and so arguably would leave the judges none the wiser. In order to resolve this issue, we must look briefly into the debate about permanence and irreversibility.

We should begin by recognizing a very important, but often neglected, point. Human beings have been dying for 200,000 years. Although the ideas of an afterlife and bringing people back from the dead are old, the concept of resuscitation medicine is relatively new, dating back only 200–300 years. Bringing someone back from the *dead* is not the same as resuscitation because the latter involves *keeping someone alive* whereas the former means bringing someone back from *death*. Contemporary debates in medicine and bioethics about the definition of death are ensconced in presuppositions about the achievements of modern technology and developments in the ICU, but it is important to take a wider, 'genealogical' look at the concept of death in order to understand modern death declaration practice and the endorsement of permanence over irreversibility.

As mentioned already, before the advent of modern resuscitative technology and the ICU, the main issues in death declaration practice concerned timeliness and safety of diagnosis, and the fact that these twin requirements might seem to pull in different directions. Fears of premature burial meant that we needed to be certain that death had occurred, and signs of putrefaction yielded this certainty. But waiting for putrefaction compromised the timeliness requirement. It is in this context that Eugène Bouchut won the Academy of Sciences prize—he offered the best compromise between safety and timeliness.

The crucial point is that Bouchut's method of declaring death is still widely used today in modern hospital practice. If the only literature a reader is familiar with is the bioethical debate on the definition of death, the continued use of the stethoscope in death declaration practice today would seem immensely puzzling. How can it be that death can still be declared once the heart stops when we could massage the heart and potentially resuscitate people for periods significantly in excess of any five-minute time frame? This puzzle dissolves, however, when we remember that, in the vast majority of death diagnoses, it will not be appropriate to attempt any form of resuscitation. In most cases, Bouchut's stethoscope remains appropriate, because resuscitation is not an option and there is accordingly no need to wait for the amount of time that would need to pass if resuscitative measures were to be attempted and fail before we could declare death.

Some bioethicists remain puzzled by this. Why can some patients be declared dead in five minutes if they are not going to receive CPR, but not if they do? These bioethicists claim that the time at which someone must have died should surely be the same for all patients.[67] The difficulty with this view is that it ignores the fact that, even on the irreversibility criterion, the time at which someone's circulation irreversibly ceases can vary from individual to individual. Nobody actually knows the point at which a person's cessation of circulation becomes irreversible. Different candidate time frames have been suggested, ranging from a few minutes to 'several hours'.[68] Theoretically, therefore, by using extracorporeal membrane oxygenation (ECMO), the circulation could be started in patients who are undergoing rigor mortis, even though we would never dream of trying. The only reason we do not do this is that it would be inappropriate to do so given the damage that the brain would have sustained by this time.

It seems, therefore, that both the advocates of the five-minute permanent standard and the advocates of the irreversible standard are actually relying on the permanence standard to declare death, because they both rely on the inappropriateness of certain measures to declare death when they do. When there is a 'do not attempt resuscitation' (DNAR) order, it is not ethically appropriate to attempt any form of resuscitation, because doing so would be battery. Likewise, one does not need to try ECMO resuscitation (or prolonged CPR) if it is not ethically appropriate—owing to the expected brain outcome.

Of course, being worthwhile and ethically appropriate is one thing, and being physiologically possible is quite another.[69] To wait until it is physiologically impossible to restore the circulation in all known patients would entail that we should wait many hours before we can legitimately and accurately declare death in any patient. Suppose society wanted this. Then, in that case, we would have to wait at least up until the point at which there can be no chance that ECMO would be successful in any patient before we could declare death. The immediate impact would be that in an ICU we would need to delay moving the patient to the mortuary, and the timing and nature of family grieving would alter. The times of death in police reports, and other practices such as warm autopsies, would also have to change.

There is also a further problem with the option of waiting many hours before claiming that someone has truly died. ECMO is our current most advanced resuscitation tool. But what if our technology advances again? Consider cryopreserved individuals. How should these individuals be categorized?[70] They are considered dead today, but potentially revivable in the future with the advent of new technology. This example does not just refer to a mere logical possibility, such as the possibility that you could wave a magic wand and someone could revive. A court of law has recently ordered the cryopreservation of the body of a 14-year-old girl suffering from incurable cancer, agreeing that it is possible that technology could one day be able not only to cure the cancer she has but also to revive her.[71] Yet the cryopreservation that took place here is a post-mortem procedure. The 14-year-old girl died first and only then was cryopreserved. Society would likely decide later, if the technology were truly realised, that this girl was dead and brought back to life, which would allow us to continue to describe the cryopreservation of this girl as a post-mortem procedure.[72] However, on the option we are now considering (waiting until we can be sure that a patient is irreversible before declaring death), we could never really know that it was actually a post-mortem procedure. Whether it was or not would be entirely dependent on what happens in the future. On the irreversibility proponents' view, we might be wrong that this girl was cryopreserved after her death (rather than before it). We are not in a position to know for certain that she is dead because, if this girl were brought back to life, then we would have discovered that, contrary to what we had all assumed, she was always alive.[73]

Does this mean we could never really be sure when someone is dead unless putrefaction has started to occur (putrefaction would mean that cryopreservation would be impossible)? If so, this position potentially takes us back to death declaration practices that were prevalent before the advent of modern medicine.[74] We doubt very much that many bioethicists, or society at large, would want to accept the claim that we can never really be sure that, at the time we currently declare death on the irreversibility criterion, it has really occurred. But, more importantly, it would mean that the point at which someone is dead would itself, once again, depend on our practices, including the practice of not cryopreserving people (because we *do* know that cryopreservation and later revival are only possible if cryopreservation is performed very quickly after death diagnosis, so, as long as we have waited long enough, we can then declare death). If making the time of death dependent on our practices seems reasonable in the case of not cryopreserving people, then on the very same logic the practice of not waiting for more than five minutes following asystole, in cases where resuscitation is not appropriate, is also reasonable.

Another objection might be that it is part of the meaning of death that it be irreversible. But this is not the case. If it were, then it would mean that bringing someone back to life would be as logically impossible as a square circle, but this doesn't appear to be right. It is also not a requirement of related concepts, such as the concept of *extinction*. If, as per Jurassic Park, we could bring back certain dinosaurs, this would not mean that they were never extinct, and that we have been wrong all this time in believing them to be extinct. We can similarly claim that if we brought someone back to life with new technology, this need not mean that they were never dead to begin with.[a] The same argument, of course, applies to permanence as to irreversibility, but the point is that there seems to be some limited wriggle room in how we use the concept of death that allows society to use it as we currently do in modern death declaration practice. Such practice relies on permanence rather than irreversibility—doctors do not routinely wait for irreversibility.[75]

Returning to the continued use of the stethoscope and Bouchut's five-minute time frame for declaring death, it is important to recognize that modern resuscitation practice became grafted on, so to speak, a century of practice which, for the vast majority of cases, it was appropriate to continue. Resuscitation would only disturb the practice recommended by Bouchut if resuscitation were appropriate for everyone, rather than for a minority of patients. And that is exactly as it should be.

The medical circulatory criteria form a halfway house between two extremes: the extreme of laypersons (and some resuscitation researchers such as Sam Parnia[76]), where someone ultimately saved from cardiac arrest can claim that they died three times on the way to hospital, and the extreme of irreversibility, where even the 97-year-old frail lady declared dead in the nursing home is not really known to be dead until several hours have passed following asystole or ECMO CPR has been attempted and failed. Such a halfway house seems an eminently reasonable compromise that continues to serve doctors and society well. There is nothing inherently wrong in diagnosing death on the basis of permanence rather than irreversibility. The Academy of Paris prize to Eugène Bouchut has stood the test of time.

Not dead—religious and conscientious objection

Families sometimes provide religious objections to stopping mechanical ventilation. In patients who have been diagnosed deceased using neurological criteria, this can be because the family do not accept that death has occurred. Some of these cases end up in the courts. It should be noted at the outset that

---

[a] It might be thought that extinction is different because we are not bringing back the same individuals whereas reviving a dead person would mean bringing back the same individual. Although true, this point is irrelevant. 'Extinction' applies to the species, 'death' to the individual, and our point is that just as, if we could revive the species, this need not mean that the revived species had never become extinct, so, if we revive an individual (for example, if they had been cryopreserved after death until new technology could revive them), this need not mean that the individual had never died.

nearly every country with advanced intensive care infrastructure accepts death using neurological criteria (even if there are some variations in the criteria) as death, including countries with strong religiosity, although the justifications can be very different (for example, Ireland and Italy—Christian; Saudi Arabia and Iran—Muslim; India—Hindu Israel—Judaism).[77,78] However, in a plural society, should greater allowance be made for religious and conscientious objection? Some have claimed so.[79,80,81,82]

In general terms, and this is an area of considerable debate and challenge, four different societal positions have been taken (see Box 7.2).

In 2015, a case came to the English court where the father asked the court to decide if brainstem death was synonymous with clinical death.[83] The family was Muslim and the father did not consider the two to be equivalent. The precedent for accepting brainstem death as death in the UK is well established.[84,85] It is, therefore, of no surprise that the Honourable Mr. Justice Hayden ruled that '[w]hilst expressing profound respect for the father's views, the time has now come to permit the ventilator to be turned off and to allow Child A, who died on 10 February, dignity in death.'[86] A different case has recently been tested in the Court of Appeal and the diagnosis once again was upheld.[87] The current position in the UK is that the diagnosis of death using neurological criteria is legal death and there is no right to conscientious objection.

Box 7.2. Four positions society has adopted to religious and conscientious objection to death diagnosed using neurological criteria

---

1. The diagnosis of death using neurological criteria is legal death and there can be *no conscientious objection* (the UK position).
2. The diagnosis of death using neurological criteria is legal death but *what the family choose to do with the body of the deceased*, including continuing mechanical ventilation, *is their concern*, provided it is privately funded (the case of Jahi McMath is an example).
3. There is *allowance for conscientious objection*, by individuals or families on the individual's behalf, to a diagnosis of death using neurological criteria being legal death (the New Jersey position and what plaintiffs in Canada are requesting).
4. *Individuals must choose, in advance*, whether or not to accept the diagnosis of death using neurological criteria as legal death (arguably the Japanese position).

The case of Jahi McMath is arguably the most controversial and well-known case of family objection to death using neurological criteria in recent years.[88,89] Jahi was a 13-year-old girl who suffered hypoxic brain injury after elective tonsil surgery. She was diagnosed deceased using neurological criteria on 12 December 2013. Her family objected to the diagnosis on a number of grounds and have claimed subsequently that her limb movements, available to view on YouTube, are proof of Jahi's conscious awareness rather than the well-described sign of spinal reflexes. Leaving aside objections on diagnostic grounds, Jahi's family have also objected on the basis of their Christian faith.[90] What is unusual in Jahi's case is that, although the Californian courts upheld the diagnosis of death as legal death (which the family continue to contest), the custody of Jahi's body was given over to her family. With donated financial support, her family moved Jahi to New Jersey. Eventually, Jahi was moved into private accommodation with her family, while still on mechanical ventilation. This remained the case until she developed excessive bleeding and liver failure, and permanent cardiac asystole occurred on 22 June 2018, nearly five years after her diagnosis of death.

It was no accident that Jahi's family moved her to New Jersey. The New Jersey Declaration of Death Act 1991 incorporates the UDDA but has some additional features, including a provision which states:

> ... if the physician has a reason to believe on the basis of information in the individual's available medical records or information provided by the family or others that the individual's personal religious beliefs would be violated by the declaration of death upon the basis of the neurological criteria, then the death of the individual shall be declared, and the time of death fixed, solely upon the basis of cardio-respiratory criteria.[91]

New York similarly allows for the 'reasonable accommodation of the individual's religious or moral objection to the determination as expressed by the individual, or by the next of kin or other person closest to the individual'.[92] This provision is written into the Codes, Rules and Regulations of the New York Department of Health, rather than primary legislation.

At the time of writing, there were two cases in the Canadian courts where families are claiming a right to religious freedom and that this should include the right to conscientiously object to the diagnosis of death using neurological criteria. This legal claim is based on the *Charter of Rights and Freedoms*, as written into the Canadian constitution, and which grants individuals in Canada the right to 'freedom of conscious and religion', 'the right to life liberty and security of the person' and to be protected from religious discrimination.[93] The first case of Shalom Ouanounou concerned a 25-year-old orthodox Jew in Toronto intubated for an asthma attack on 27 September 2017, declared deceased using neurological criteria and who eventually developed permanent cardiac asystole in March 2018 after five months in hospital.[94] His family pursued a legal challenge, without success, even after Shalom's funeral. The second case from Canada concerned the case of 27-year-old Taquisha McKitty who suffered an out-of-hospital cardiac arrest and whose death was diagnosed using neurological criteria in September 2017.[95] Taquisha's family objected to her diagnosis of death on the grounds that she was not dead according to the laws and precepts of her Christian faith. Justice Lucille Shaw, in the Ontario Superior Court of Justice, concluded that 'brain death extinguishes personhood, and with it, the right to assert *Charter* protection'.[96] Taquisha developed permanent cardiac asystole in December 2018, after the Court of Appeal had heard her case but before its judgement. The Court, as expected, ruled that the diagnosis of death using neurological criteria was legal death, but chose not to rule on whether a religious objection was permissible on the grounds the case was moot, owing to Taquisha now satisfying both neurological and circulatory criteria for death.[97]

The situation in Japan is unique, reflecting perhaps a long ambivalence to death diagnosed using neurological criteria.[98] The specific wording in Japan's Organ Transplant Law in 1997 can be read as implying an allowance for people to decide in advance whether neurological criteria can be used to determine their death.[99] Whether a person was dead using neurological criteria depended on what was going to occur afterwards—namely, if the individual had followed Japan's very strict opt-in policy and had given written consent in advance for organ donation and there was no family veto.[100] So, only if the person chose to be a donor after death could a diagnosis of death using neurological criteria be made. Even with a revision of the law in 2009 to an opt-out system, it has not entirely removed the debate of whether neurological criteria can be applied regardless of organ donation concerns.[101,102] This reflects the ambiguity that will occur if legal definitions of death exist only as part of transplant law, rather than law applicable to every member of society.

Conscientious objection raises extremely difficult and contentious issues. On the one hand, we tend to consider death to be an objective matter of fact, like the boiling point of water (given certain constant background conditions). Someone is either alive or dead, in the same way that water is either boiling or it is not. The argument would be that, just as we could not plausibly allow conscientious objection about the boiling point of water, so we cannot plausibly allow conscientious objection about the point at which someone is dead. Nonetheless, the case of death is more complicated because genuine conceptual questions are raised about what should count as a human being's having died in the wake of certain technological developments (see page X). If, as we have seen, there are cases where we may need to stipulate a new definition or use of a term, then there may be cases where several *reasonable* options are open in terms of how society should alter a concept (several reasonable stipulations being in the offing). If that is so, then the one chosen by the medical profession and lawmakers may not be the same option as that which would be chosen by some religious leaders and religious people who have firm beliefs about what should be required before death can be declared.

In this situation, we believe the question is whether allowing conscientious objection to accommodate these different views would have a detrimental effect on public confidence in death declaration practice. There is no doubt room for ongoing debate about this, but there is another issue here that we should consider and which might make the concern about public confidence especially pressing. As Dominic Wilkinson has suggested,[103] it is difficult to restrict conscientious objection simply to beliefs stemming from religious creeds and practice. What if some objections come from *secular* quarters? Some people might disagree with the options chosen by the medical profession as a whole and law makers, without that objection stemming from any religious beliefs. It is difficult to claim that these objections should not be accommodated, and that only the religious ones should be. Ethically, the *source* of the objection does not seem to be relevant to its *content*. However, once we allow anyone to object on the basis of their personal beliefs, the risk of public confidence in death declaration practice being undermined surely increases: having different standards or definitions of death, with no restrictions on the circumstances in which such different standards or definitions can be acknowledged, is liable to invite confusion about death and undermine many of the practices that are based on it. For this reason, it might be preferable to favour the approach taken by UK courts, that there is no right of conscientious objection.

Conclusion

It was societal forces that established a duty upon doctors to diagnose death. Medical advances over the past two centuries have challenged our definitions and criteria and caused them to evolve. This trend continues. Head transplants may seem like science fiction, but history has shown that such fiction becomes science more quickly than one expects. The need then for doctors, willing to fulfil their societal duty of being safe and timely in the diagnosis of death, will continue. Perhaps all one can conclude is that it was very lucky for Harry Potter that Lord Voldemort sent Narcissa Malfoy to see if he was dead; had he sent a doctor, the outcome would have been very different.

References

1. Powner D, Ackerman B, Grenvik A. (1996) Medical diagnosis of death in adults: historical contributions to current controversies. *Lancet* 348:1219–23.
2. Trubuhovich R. (2007) History of mouth-to-mouth ventilation. Part 3: the 19th to mid-20th centuries and 'rediscovery'. *Critical Care and Resuscitation* 9(2):221–37.
3. Safar P. (1989) History of cardio-pulmonary-cerebral resuscitation. In: Kaye W, Bircher NG. (eds) *Clinics in critical care medicine: cardiopulmonary resuscitation.* Churchill Livingston Inc., New York.
4. Bondeson J. (2002) *Buried alive: the terrifying history of our most primal fear.* W.W. Norton, London.
5. Lear T. (1799) The diary account: the last illness and death of General Washington. https://founders.archives.gov/documents/Washington/06-04-02-0406-0002 (accessed 5 December 2019).
6. Tebb W, Vollum EP, Hadwen WR. (2012) *Premature burial: how it may be prevented.* Jonathan Sale (ed). First published 1905. National Press, Jordan.
7. Bouchut, E. (1849) Traité des signes de la mort et des moyens de prévenir les enterrements prématurés [online]. https://archive.org/details/traitdessignes00bouc (accessed 5 December 2019).
8. Ibid.
9. Mollaret P, Goulon M. (1959) Le coma de´passe´ depassed coma (me´moire pre´liminaire). *Revue Neurologique (Paris)* 101:3–15.
10. Ad hoc committee of the Harvard Medical School (1968). A definition of irreversible coma. Report of the ad hoc committee of the Harvard Medical School to examine the definition of brain death. *Journal of the American Medical Association* 205:337–40.
11. Belkin GS. (2014) *Death before dying. History, medicine and brain death.* Oxford University Press.
12. Ibid.
13. Machado C, Korein J, Ferrer T, et al. (2007) The declaration of Sydney on human death. *Journal of Medical Ethics* 33:699–703.
14. Honorary secretary (1976) Diagnosis of brain death. Statement issued by the honorary secretary of the Conference of Medical Royal Colleges and their Faculties in the United Kingdom on 11 October 1976. *British Medical Journal* 6045:1187–8.

15. Honorary secretary (1979) Diagnosis of death. Memorandum issued by the honorary secretary of the Conference of Medical Royal Colleges and their Faculties in the United Kingdom on 15 January 1979. *British Medical Journal* 6159:332.

16. Academy of Medical Royal Colleges (2008) *A code of practice for the diagnosis and confirmation of death*. Academy of Medical Royal Colleges. London. http://aomrc. org.uk/wp-content/uploads/2016/04/Code_Practice_Confirmation_Diagnosis_ Death_1008-4.pdf (accessed 9 December 2019).

17. National Conference of Commissioners on Uniform State Laws (1981) Uniform determination of death act [online]. https://www.uniformlaws.org/HigherLogic/ System/DownloadDocumentFile.ashx?DocumentFileKey=341343fa-1efe-706c-043a-9290fdcfd909&forceDialog=0 (accessed 21 December 2019).

18. The President's Council on Bioethics (2008) *Controversies in the determination of death: a white paper by the president's council on bioethics.* http://bioethics.georgetown.edu/pcbe/reports/death/ (accessed 5 December 2019).

19. Ibid.

20. Bernat JL, Capron AM, Bleck TP, et al. (2010) The circulatory–respiratory determination of death in organ donation. *Critical Care Medicine* 38:963–70.

21. Safar, History of cardio-pulmonary-cerebral resuscitation.

22. Shemie SD, Hornby L, Baker A, et al. (2014) International guideline development for the determination of death. *Intensive Care Medicine* 40(6):788–97.

23. Shemie S, Gardiner D. (2018) Circulatory arrest, brain arrest and death determination. *Frontiers in Cardiovascular Medicine* 5:15. doi: 10.3389/fcvm.2018.00015. (accessed 5 December 2019).

24. Gardiner D, Shemie S, Manara A, Opdam H. (2012) International perspective on the diagnosis of death. *British Journal of Anaesthesia* 108 Suppl 1:i14–28.

25. Ibid.

26. Green MB, Wikler D. (1980) Brain death and personal identity. *Philosophy and Public Affairs* 9:105–33.

27. Monti MM, Vanhaudenhuyse A, Coleman MR, et al. (2010) Willful modulation of brain activity in disorders of consciousness. *New England Journal of Medicine* 362:579–89.

28. Machado C, Estevez M, Rodriguez R, et al. (2016) Vegetative state and the other world. In: Leisman G, Merrick J. (eds) *Functional neurology: considering consciousness clinically.* Nova Science Publishers, New York: 99–120.

29. Posner JB, Plum F. (2007) Pathophysiology of signs and symptoms of coma. In: Posner JB, Saper CB, Schiff ND, Plum F. (eds) Plum and Posner's diagnosis of stupor and coma, 4th edn. Oxford University Press: 3–37.

30. President's Council, *Controversies in the determination of death.*

31. Gardiner et al., International perspective on the diagnosis of death.

32. Shewmon A. (1998) Chronic 'brain death: meta-analysis and conceptual consequences.' *Neurology* 51:1538–45.

33. Shewmon A. (2009) Brain death: can it be resuscitated? *Hastings Center Report* 39(2):18–24.

34. Nair-Collins M. (2010) Death, brain death, and the limits of science. *Journal of Law, Medicine and Ethics* 38(3):667–83.

35. Miller F, Truog R. (2012) *Death, dying and organ transplantation: reconstructing medical ethics and the end of life.* Oxford University Press.

36. Bernat JL. (2008) Brain death. In: Bernat JL, Ethical issues in neurology. Lippincott Williams & Wilkins: Philadelphia: 253–86.

37. Lee P. (2016) Total brain death and the integration of the body required of a human being. *Journal of Medicine and Philosophy* 41(3):300–14.

38. Moschella M. (2016) Integrated but not whole? Applying an ontological account of human organismal unity to the brain death debate. *Bioethics* 30(8):550–6.

39. Machado et al., The declaration of Sydney on human death.

40. Lamba N, Holsgrove D, Broekman M. (2016) The history of head transplantation: a review. *Acta Neurochirurgica* 158:2239–47.

41. McGee A. (2016) We are human beings. *Journal of Medicine and Philosophy* 41:148–71.

42. Glock HJ. (1996) *A Wittgenstein dictionary.* Blackwell, Oxford.

43. National Conference of Commissioners of Uniform State Lawyers, Uniform Determination of Death Act.

44. Academy of Medical Royal Colleges, *A code of practice.*

45. Shemie et al., International guideline development.

46. Gardiner et al., International perspective on the diagnosis of death.

47. Wijdicks EF, Varelas PN, Gronseth GS, Greer DM. (2010) Evidence-based guideline update: determining brain death in adults: report of the Quality Standards Subcommittee of the American Academy of Neurology. *Neurology* 74:1911–18.

48. Varelas PN, Brady P, Rehman M, Afshinnik A, Mehta C, Abdelhak T, Wijdicks EF. (2017) Primary posterior fossa lesions and preserved supratentorial cerebral blood flow: implications for brain death determination. *Neurocritical Care* 27(3):407–14.

49. President's Council, *Controversies in the determination of death.*

50. Daniel PM. (1966) The blood supply of the hypothalamus and pituitary gland. *British Medical Bulletin* 22:202.

51. Nussey S, Whitehead S. (2001) The pituitary gland. In: Nussey S, Whitehead S, eds, Endocrinology: an integrated approach. BIOS Scientific Publishers, Oxford. http://www.ncbi.nlm.nih.gov/books/NBK27/#A1297 (accessed 5 December 2019).

52. Dalle Ave AL, Bernat JL. (2018) Inconsistencies between the criterion and tests for brain death. *Journal of Intensive Care Medicine.* doi: 10.1177/0885066618784268.

53. Pope TM. (2018) Brain death forsaken: growing conflict and new legal challenges. *Journal of Legal Medicine* 37:265–324.

54. Ahmed F, Tabassum N, Rasool S. (2012) Regulation of atrial natriuretic peptide (ANP) and its role in blood pressure. *International Current Pharmaceutical Journal* 1(7):176–9.

55. McGee A, Gardiner D. (2018) Differences in the definition of brain death and their legal impact on intensive care practice. *Anaesthesia* doi:10.1111/anae.14568.

56. Truog R, Miller F. (2010) Counterpoint: are donors after circulatory death really dead, and does it matter? No, and not really. *Chest* 138:16–18.

57. Joffe AR, Carcillo J, Anton N, deCaen A, Han YY, Bell MJ, Maffei FA, Sullivan J, Thomas J, Garcia-Guerra G. (2011) Donation after cardiocirculatory death: a call for a moratorium pending full public disclosure and fully informed consent. *Philosophy, Ethics, and Humanities in Medicine* 6:17.

58. Miller et al., *Death, dying and organ transplantation.*

59. Truog et al., Counterpoint.

60. Marquis D. (2010) Are DCD donors really dead? *Hastings Center Report* 40(3):24–31.

61. McGee A, Gardiner D. (2017) Permanence can be defended. *Bioethics* 31(3):220–30.

62. McGee A, Gardiner D. (2018) Donation after the circulatory determination of death: some responses to recent criticisms. *The Journal of Medicine and Philosophy* 43:211–40.

63. McGee A, Gardiner D, Murphy P. (2018) Determination of death in donation after circulatory death: an ethical propriety. *Current Opinion in Organ Transplantation* 23(1):114–19.

64. National Conference of Commissioners of Uniform State Lawyers, Uniform Determination of Death Act.

65. Gardiner D, Housley G, Shaw D. (2016) Diagnosis of death in modern hospital practice. In: Leisman G, Merrick J, (eds) *Functional Neurology: Considering Consciousness Clinically.* Nova Science Publishers: New York: 93–7.

66. National Conference of Commissioners of Uniform State Lawyers, Uniform Determination of Death Act.

67. McGee et al., Donation after the circulatory determination of death.

68. DeVita, M. (2001) The death watch: certifying death using cardiac criteria. *Progress in Transplantation* 11(1):58–66.

69. Marquis, Are DCD donors really dead?

70. Shaw D. (2009) Cryoethics: seeking life after death. *Bioethics* 23(9):515–21.

71. BBC News (2016) Terminally ill teen won historic ruling to preserve body. https://www.bbc.co.uk/news/health-38012267 (accessed 5 December 2019).

72. McGee et al., Permanence can be defended.

73. Joffe A. (2018) DCDD Donors are not dead. *Hastings Center Report:* doi.org/10.1002/hast.949 (accessed 5 December 2019).

74. McGee et al., Donation after the circulatory determination of death.

75. Gardiner et al., Diagnosis of death in modern hospital practice.

76. Parnia S (2013) The Lazarus Effect. Random House: London.

77. EF. Wijdicks (2002) Brain death worldwide accepted fact but no global consensus in diagnostic criteria. *Neurology* 58(1):20–5.

78. Aramesh K, Arima H, Gardiner D, Sham SK. (2018) An international legal review of the relationship between brain death and organ transplantation. *Journal of Clinical Ethics* 29(1):31–42.

79. Veatch RM. (1999) The conscious clause: how much individual choice in defining death can our society tolerate? In: Younger SJ, Arnold RM, Schapiro R. (eds) The *definition of death—contemporary controversies.* The John Hopkins University Press: Baltimore.

80. Olick RS, Braun EA, Potash J. (2009) Accommodating religious and moral objections to neurological death. *The Journal of Clinical Ethics* 20(2):183–91.

81. Choong KA. (2013) Organ procurement: a case for pluralism on the definition of death. *Journal of Medical Law and Ethics* 1:5–21.

82. Johnson LSM. (2016) The case for reasonable accommodation of conscientious objections to declarations of brain death. *Journal of Bioethical Inquiry* 13(1):105–15.

83. Re A (A Child) [2015] EWHC 443 (Fam).

84. Re: A (A Minor) [1992] 3 Medical Law Reports 303.

85. Re: TC (A Minor) [1994], 2 Medical Law Review 376.

86. Re A (A Child) [2015] EWHC 443 (Fam).

87. [2020] EWCA Civ 164 https://www.judiciary.uk/judgments/re-m-declaration-of-death-of-child/ (accessed 28 February 2020).

88. Pope, Brain death forsaken.

89. Truog RD. (2018) Defining death—making sense of the case of Jahi McMath. *Journal of the American Medical Association* 319:1859–60.

90. Johnson, The Case for Reasonable Accommodation.

91. Brown ML. (2013) State of New Jersey. New Jersey law revision commission. Draft final report. Relating to New Jersey Declaration of Death Act. http://www.lawrev.state.nj.us/UDDA/njddaDFR010713.pdf (accessed 5 December 2019).

92. New York Department of Health (2018) 10 CRR-NY 400.16 Determination of death. https://govt.westlaw.com/nycrr/Document/I4fe2fa1dcd1711dda432a117e6e0f345?viewType=FullText&originationContext=documenttoc&transitionType=CategoryPageItem&contextData=(sc.Default) (accessed 5 December 2019).

93. Government of Canada (2018) Guide to the Canadian Charter of Rights and Freedoms. https://www.canada.ca/en/canadian-heritage/services/how-rights-protected/guide-canadian-charter-rights-freedoms.html#a2b (accessed 5 December 2019).

94. McGillivray, K. (2018) Jewish man at the centre of religious debate to be remembered at funeral. https://www.cbc.ca/news/canada/toronto/shalom-ouanounou-death-1.4569257 (accessed 5 December 2019).

95. Justice Shaw. (2018) McKitty v Hayani ONSC 4015, [53]. https://www.canlii.org/en/on/onsc/doc/2018/2018onsc4015/2018onsc4015.pdf (accessed 5 December 2019).

96. Ibid.

97. McKitty v. Hayani, 2019 ONCA805.

98. Lock MM. (2002) *Twice dead: organ transplants and the reinvention of death.* University of California Press: Berkeley.

99. Bagheri A. (2007) Individual choice in the definition of death. *Journal of Medical Ethics* 33(3):146–9.

100. Aramesh et al., An international legal review.

101. Ibid.

102. Choong, Organ procurement.

103. Wilkinson, D. (2017) Conscientious non-objection in intensive care. *Cambridge Quarterly of Healthcare Ethics* **26**: 132–42.

PART C

EXTERNAL INFLUENCES

8

Doing What's Best

Organ Donation and Intensive Care

Louise Austin and John Coggon

Introduction

This chapter goes to the core of an area of ongoing controversy in the critical care community.[1,2,3,4,5] It examines the effect of the best interests standard on decisions relating to patients in intensive care who physically would be appropriate candidates for organ donation. The particular focus is on controlled non-heart-beating organ donation (NHBOD), whereby organ retrieval takes place following the planned withdrawal of life support, and thus when the time of cardiac death is controlled.[a] We begin by acknowledging the concerns that healthcare professionals might feel, before providing an analysis of medical law as it relates to decision making. Exploration and understanding of legal principle allow us to provide an account of good practice in decision making in this context. We set aside illusory concerns, and bring to the fore the key matters that the law demands be considered by decision makers.

We conclude that the law on best interests must not be subjected to the narrow simplification that has in the past beset it. As best interests demands that due account be given to patients' moral, social, ethical, religious, and other values and beliefs, it is wrong to believe that a treatment decision can be based on an assessment purely of clinical benefits, or on a fictitiously atomized view of the patient. We therefore argue that there will be many situations where controlled NHBOD will be in the best interests of patients in intensive care. Our view is supported by the Department of Health's 2009 guidance[10] but, despite this and our certainty about the case we make, we recognize that there are continued concerns from practitioners and academics. Some of these concerns, as they relate to our argument, are addressed within this chapter. We would, however, urge the General Medical Council to follow the Department

---

[a] It builds upon and reflects arguments previously made by Coggon and colleagues.[6,7,8,9]

of Health's approach by providing greater reassurance and clarity in its advice to practitioners than is the case in its current guidance.[11] The chapter ends with a brief consideration of the lack of legal certainty regarding the necessary observation time between the cessation of heart beat and the commencement of organ retrieval.

The apparent minefield

Medical practice, it might be argued, would be a lot easier if there were no lawyers standing on the sidelines waiting to declare what is right or wrong in a given situation. Healthcare law and ethics has greatly expanded as an academic field, as well as an area of perennial interest to the press, parliament, and pressure groups. Throughout the literature—public and academic—divergent views abound concerning what is proper practice. It would be no surprise, therefore, if practitioners were to feel that perhaps they would be best off working under an exacting version of the 'precautionary principle'. But even trying to work in accordance with precaution is hard: it is often not clear what the most conservative course of action might be. The practice of so-called 'defensive medicine' is well recognized and easily put down in texts such as this.[b] It can at times be harder, however, to persuade physicians of what is acceptable, lawful practice. This is particularly so in relation to areas of profound social and ethical contention, such as organ retrieval. However, we aim here to explain and explore the correct understanding of law as it has been settled both in the courts and by Parliament, and thus provide some real reassurance to intensive care specialists about the propriety of what might seem to be a legal and ethical minefield. Our focus is on modest—but to some minds contentious—measures that may be taken in intensive care for patients who might become organ donors. We consider the prolongation of life support following a decision that *from a purely clinical perspective* continued provision of treatment is futile: controlled NHBOD. Can it be lawful to allow ventilation to persist in order that the surgical retrieval team has time to coordinate itself and be prepared to have optimal chances of a successful transplantation? We will demonstrate that, as suggested by the Department of Health's 2009 guidance,[10] the answer to this question is yes.

McGee and White argue that while the 2009 guidance states that the question of whether to prolong treatment in these circumstances is to be decided

---

[b] See Reference 12, pp. 253–5, for discussion of how much a problem defensive medicine is in practice.

independently of the question of organ donation, if facilitation of organ donation forms part of the assessment of best interests, then the two have to be considered together[13] (pp. 137–8). We believe this misunderstands the questions
the treating clinician must ask. The first question is whether treatment is clinically futile. That decision is made independently of the question of organ donation. If the clinician concludes it is futile, the next step is to assess whether,
despite the futility of the treatment, it is in the patient's best interests that it
should continue. It is at that second stage that the assessment of best interests
comes into play, which we argue (and the 2009 guidance supports) goes beyond clinical best interests and should include consideration of the patient's
wishes about organ donation.

Given the well-known scandals relating to posthumous organ retrieval,[14,15]
whose aftermath is still felt, the current position of healthcare practitioners at-
tracts some sympathy: there are radically competing views that proliferate in
the literature, both regarding the law and the ethics of organ donation. Bell, a
clinician who has published repeatedly on the subject, states that '[T]here are
salient ethical, legal and logistical hurdles to defensible introduction of either
controlled or uncontrolled NHBOD . . . '[16] (p. 825).

What, then, are physicians to do? On the one hand, many will be acutely
aware of the mismatch between the numbers of people who say they would
be willing to donate organs after death and those who actually do.[17] On the
other hand, many practitioners will be afraid of potential legal ramifications
(not to mention ethical criticism or even scandal) if they appear to harm a
patient's autonomy or bodily integrity in order to optimize the opportunities
for donation. At the time of writing, the English legal position does not base
itself on a presumption that a person would wish to donate.[18] However, following the passing of the Organ Donation (Deemed Consent) Act 2019, that
will change in spring 2020 to reflect the position in Welsh law. In Wales, a
person is deemed to have consented to organ donation unless they made a decision about organ donation before their death, or appointed a person to make
such decisions on their behalf.[19] Yet in the case of an incapacitated person, the
Welsh Act provides that if, for a significant period before their death, the deceased person lacked the capacity to understand the effect of deemed consent,
then the deemed consent provisions will not apply (s.5(3)(b)). The English
Act also adopts this position (s.1). The adoption of deemed consent to posthumous organ donation in England will not, however, resolve the question
of whether it is lawful to prolong treatment of an incapacitated person to facilitate organ recovery: moving to a system of presumed consent to posthumous organ donation does not, of itself, speak to the lawfulness of premortem
interventions.

So what is a doctor to do when a living patient, who lacks capacity and is inevitably close to death, may be a suitable donor? Is there a clash in duties, and, if so, which duty prevails? Can it be lawful to base treatment options for the patient on potential benefit to a third party? In what follows, we explore these and related questions. By understanding the law's demands regarding medical decision making, it will become clear that decisions can be made to treat a patient in a way that will benefit a third party. In other words, for a patient who lacks capacity to consent, it can be lawful to undertake harmless acts that enhance the chances of successful organ retrieval, even when these acts confer no *clinical* benefit to the patient who will become a posthumous donor.

The good, the bad, and the clinical

If we could all agree on what is good and what is bad, decision making would be a great deal less contentious. But life is not so simple, and the law is not either. A liberal social system recognizes that a plurality of views exists, and in many circumstances the default position at law is that the views on what is best should be left to the individual. However, this position is necessarily qualified in various ways. As is familiar in a healthcare context, medical expertise will only be deferred to if it is supported by a responsible body of medical opinion.[20,21] And if we take the paradigm case of a competent, adult patient, the decision-making capacity given to them is tempered by limits on their positive freedoms. The freedom from interference—sometimes called the 'right to bodily integrity'—is absolute: the patient can say 'no' to any interference proposed as being to their benefit. The strength of this right is often emphasized through expression of Lord Donaldson MR's celebrated dictum in the case of *Re T* that a person is free to refuse a medical intervention for any reason, be it 'rational, irrational, unknown or even non-existent'[22] (p. 102). And this is reinforced by the principle found in the Mental Capacity Act 2005, section 1(4): 'A person is not to be treated as unable to make a decision merely because he makes an unwise decision.'

We shall consider this further later, but should note here that one interpretation of the legal position is that the law is indifferent to the well-being of adult patients who have capacity: the law demands that you leave alone such a patient who refuses treatment, even if they appear to be harming themselves by doing this. They could tell you they have no reason to be harming themselves, or even that their reason is that Tuesday begins with a W, and still you would have to leave them alone. Were they without capacity, you would treat them in their best interests, but until the presumption of capacity is rebutted you have to watch them suffer. Thus, are we to be unconcerned by the best interests of apparently unwise decision makers? Arguably, the answer to this is no: that we are not disregarding their best interests by accepting their refusal of consent. The law's emphasis on not questioning a decision because of its apparent lack of wisdom is a means of avoiding value despotism. As an individual is sovereign, at least of their negative freedom, the law cannot allow government to be transferred to a third party. Thus, the respect demanded by law for an adult's right to refuse rests on a need for due deference to the individual's self-government rather than a need to endorse (or approve of, or agree with) the individual's conclusions on what best serves them.[c] As the law works to preserve value pluralism, a strong, overarching conception of the good cannot trump every arguably bad choice a person makes. As such a system is conducive to the well-being of individuals, and recognizes that opinions validly differ,[d] the law's apparent indifference to a patient's irrational or baseless refusal in itself serves their interests, rather than harms them.[e]

If we move to consider positive freedom—'freedom *to*' as opposed to 'freedom *from*'[26]—the individual's powers of self-government cannot be described as absolute. Here the law has a more defensible role in defining benefit and harm. Once people are involved in social interactions, especially those involving state actors (such as doctors working for the National Health Service), it would be unsustainable for individuals to have absolute rights to demand whatever treatment they thought was suitable. In situations where positive demands are made, standards imposed by value systems external to the patient's own come into play. So, while an adult with capacity does not need their doctor to agree that they should *refuse* treatment for some reason, they cannot expect their doctor to agree that they should *receive* any treatment for any reason.[f]

The crux of this is not on an overall 'life view', or an all-things-considered assessment of good and bad. Rather, it swings on the issue of clinical interests, or what may be labelled the '*Bolam* aspect' of the decision. The law recognizes a patient's right to healthcare, and thus a duty on the state to provide it, but *exercise* of the right is not founded (purely, at least) on the patient's assessment of need. It is tempered necessarily by (in principle) just processes of allocation

---

[c] For an application of this, consider the case of *Ms B* (Reference 23).

[d] For an account of such liberalism, see Reference 24.

[e] For application of this in the context of competent decisions concerning posthumous organ donation, see Reference 25.

[f] For a deep, critical analysis of the ideas presented in these paragraphs, see Reference 27.

in a system supported by finite resources, and also by clinical expertise.[8] This ensures that the interests of all, and not just the individual, are served while respecting autonomy through the adoption of a relational, rather than an individualistic, approach. McLean has said that:

> [...] relational autonomy does not seek to deny the importance of decisional freedom that is so dear to the heart of individualistic autonomy. Rather, socially and politically it seeks to accommodate what are seen as reasonable (and ethically justifiable) constraints on the excessive selfishness that individualistic autonomy would, opponents say, have few, if any, means of preventing.[32] (p. 23)

Therefore, in the Court of Appeal decision in *Burke*, Lord Phillips MR held that:

> The proposition that the patient has a paramount right to refuse treatment is amply demonstrated by the authorities cited by Munby J in paragraphs 54 to 56 of his [first instance] judgement [of this case] under the heading '*Autonomy and self-determination*'. The corollary does not, however, follow, at least as a general proposition. Autonomy and the right of self-determination do not entitle the patient to insist on receiving a particular medical treatment regardless of the nature of the treatment. Insofar as a doctor has a legal obligation to provide treatment, this cannot be founded simply upon the fact that the patient demands it. The source of the duty lies elsewhere.[33] (para. 31)

As the jurisprudence on best interests and patient choice has developed, most pronouncedly in that relating to best interests, it has become clear that the law divides healthcare decision making into questions about what is clinically indicated—or at times what is clinically defensible—and what is indicated overall given all the relevant values. The resultant position is that, as Dame Elizabeth Butler-Sloss put it in *Re S*, the right decision depends not solely on an assessment defensible by reference to the *Bolam* test, but must 'incorporate broader ethical, social, moral and welfare considerations'[34] (p. 28). Patients are in a position to define what is good and bad, but not what is clinically necessary. And where serving the concepts of good and bad involves the exercise of a positive right, the state also has a legitimate role in defining what is good and what is bad.[35]

Having provided this brief theoretical overview, we will now explore the application of best interests at law, and consider the relevance of capacity and

---

[8] For discussion and exploration of the complicated theoretical issues buried in the two sentences leading to this footnote, see References 9 and 28–31).

consent in medical decision making. This involves analysis of the question of whether we care less about those who have capacity than those who do not, a question answered by consideration of how we come to assess the interests of those who are without capacity.

Is there anything special about losing capacity? Informed consent and best interests

In the previous section, we asked whether the law is indifferent to the well-being of adults who have capacity while simultaneously caring only for the best interests of adults who are deemed to lack capacity. To consider the legal effect of losing capacity, and the interests that then present themselves, let us flip the question on its head: would the law allow a patient who lacks capacity to have their right to healthcare waived (or qualified in any way) to accord with peculiar values? The short answer is yes. When taking a legal approach, we may only *think about* best interests when we are considering patients without capacity. But best interests must not be taken to represent some sort of objective, one-size-fits-all values yardstick that can be appealed to when we cannot ask someone for consent. The law's recognition of, and respect for, diversity in values extends far beyond those of people who can make a contemporaneous decision. It is for this reason that you cannot wait for a patient who is making an apparently foolish refusal of consent to lose capacity and then overrule their previously expressed will 'using' best interests. That would be *abusing* best interests. While it may be true that our evaluations of the interests of patients who lack capacity are more engaged than a capacitous patient's assessment of her own interests need be,[h] there is no reason (or freedom) to treat the values of those without capacity differently than we would the values of a patient who is not deemed to lack capacity. The patient's values are still crucial to an understanding of what is best in the circumstances. Section 4(6) of the Mental Capacity Act obliges decision makers to consider in a best interests assessment:

so far as is reasonably ascertainable –

  a the person's past and present wishes and feelings (and, in particular, any relevant written statement made by him when he had capacity),

---

[h] That is to say, the Mental Capacity Act requires decision makers who are deciding for the patient to follow specific criteria in the process of coming to the decision. The law does not impose such exacting demands on people with capacity when they are deciding for themselves.

    b the beliefs and values that would be likely to influence his decision if he had
      capacity, and
    c the other factors that he would be likely to consider if her were able to do so.

This statutory understanding of best interests leaves little—if anything—
practically different to the common law situation that preceded it. As best
interests has developed through the case law, it has become clear that a decision is neither justified simply by, nor necessarily contingent upon, there
being a clinical benefit to the patient.[36,37] The same is true for decisions concerning patients who have capacity. When there are viable options available
(including doing nothing), these will be assessed in the light of the patient's
preferences and values. In each case, the legal presumption is that the
patient's best interests, as permitted within the scheme of rationing and provision, are being served.[i] Although commentators may choose to describe
this as an 'expanded interpretation' of best interests, it should be noted that
applying it in this way is not a question of *expanding* the interpretation afforded by law. It is expanded by contrast with a narrow perspective that considers only the *Bolam* aspect of the decision. It is not, however, an expansion
of the law or of legal principle. Without controversy or complication, best
interests is a necessarily broad standard, which demands accommodation of
the patient's values broadly understood. This all means that, in some sense,
there is nothing special about losing capacity. You are still to be treated as
an individual whose interests are your own, and whose values affect the importance and desirability of any proposed option. Furthermore, this is well-
settled law, has been for some time, and is bolstered by Parliament in the
Mental Capacity Act. The principle can be demonstrated by brief reference
to the case law.

The cases of *Re F*[39] and *Re Y*[40] both provide examples of clinical benefit
not being a necessary condition for lawful procedures to take place. In *Re
F*, the courts were asked to decide whether it would be lawful to perform a
non-therapeutic sterilization on a woman with a serious mental disability, in
order that the limited freedom she enjoyed be no further narrowed for fear
of her becoming pregnant. *Re Y* concerned the question of allowing an adult
who had never had relevant decision-making capacity to be a donor of bone
marrow to her sister, whom she could not be said to know in any meaningful
sense. In both cases, it was found that the non-therapeutic interventions were
in the best interests of the patients as *overall* they would be of benefit.

---

[i] For development of this argument, see Reference 38.

Ashan v University Hospitals Leicester NHS Trust[41] provides an example of a decision where clinical benefit is not the contingent factor in a best interests assessment. Here, the patient who had lived as a devout Muslim had fallen into a persistent vegetative state. It was argued that her best interests would be served by her receiving treatment at home, rather than in a hospital setting. The treatment she was receiving raised no clinical concerns, and it was also clear that the patient would not be aware of the move. Even so, given the patient's values, it was held that her best interests required that she be taken home.

Stammers critiques reliance on *Ashan* in this context on the basis that being cared for at home is a different outcome to continued ventilation for the purposes of facilitating organ donation.[42] Rady and Verheijde also critique the use of this case and argue that it would not justify continued treatment where such treatment was inconsistent with the patient's 'values, beliefs, and rituals' around end of life care.[43] These criticisms, however, reflect a misunderstanding of the reliance on *Ashan* in this instance. It is not used within this chapter to justify the continuance of treatment itself. Instead, it is used to illustrate that the standard of best interests is broader than consideration of clinical benefits alone.

Confirmation that the best interests standard in law is not limited to clinical benefit came in *Aintree* where the Supreme Court held that when assessing a patient's best interests:

> Decision-makers must look at his welfare in the widest sense, not just medical but social and psychological […] they must try and put themselves in the place of the individual patient and ask what his attitude to the treatment is or would be likely to be; and they must consult others who are looking after him or interested in his welfare, in particular for their view of what his attitude would be.[44] (para. 39)

Equally, for patients who have capacity, clinical benefit is neither a necessary nor a sufficient condition of lawful medical intervention. So, for example, the Human Tissue Act 2004 allows live organ donation to take place. That we could choose to donate a kidney is a manifest example of our being permitted (in principle) to perform an act that confers no clinical benefit on us. Other examples of non-therapeutic interventions that adults may nonetheless receive include assisted reproduction, sterilization, and cosmetic surgery. And it is well established at common law that a healthcare team is not justified in providing unwanted treatment to a patient with capacity, even if it does so with the very best of intentions.[45] Again the Mental Capacity Act bolsters the situation, making clear that the patient who has capacity is not to be doubted for appearing to make an unwise decision.

Thus, to the extent illustrated, we can say that—in principle—welfare concerns in any healthcare setting where we see a patient who lacks capacity in contrast with one who has capacity are illusory. In both cases, the processes that the law establishes—best interests and consent—are designed to allow the decision that is best accommodated within the value systems of the particular patient, necessarily qualified by the discussion of positive and negative freedoms. Thus, even when we are making non-clinical decisions for a patient who is deemed to lack capacity we do not need (from a legal perspective) to be concerned by the patient's lack of capacity to provide informed consent. Although a decision maker must be careful in assessing the patient's values, by following the principles developed at common law, galvanized in the Mental Capacity Act and detailed in the Act's Code of Practice, they can make *any* decision regarding the welfare of a patient who lacks capacity without fear that they are 'overstepping the mark' simply by virtue of the fact that the decision is not based purely on medical factors, or that the decision takes account of the altruistic, or other-affecting values, of the patient. We are not atomized, completely separate individuals.[46,47] Although best interests must not be used to make patients who lack capacity simply a means to a further end, it is wrong falsely to accredit persons who are deemed to lack capacity with selfish, self-centred, miserly values when these do not accord with their own values. According to law, our spiritual, familial, moral, social, and ethical values survive our capacity to understand or communicate them, and the law, as we have shown, demands that decision makers for those who have lost capacity take account of these values when deciding what would be best for the patient.

Is there anything special about dying?

As we are considering the application of the best interests standard in intensive care, it might strike some that we ought to ask if there is anything special about dying that might render treatment of dying patients a 'special case'. For intuitive, emotional, or deep-seated ethical reasons, people might argue that an extraordinary level and standard of care ought to apply when we are dealing with a patient at the end of life. Simon Woods argues in favour of enhanced protection being given to an individual's perceptions of their interests as they die, in essence suggesting that we ought to enhance the freedom to act in accordance with the interests of the patient as they see them as life comes to an end.[48,49] It is likely that Munby J. was driven by some similar type of concern when handing down his (subsequently overturned) judgement in the *Burke* case.[50] Here, Munby J. found that a human 'right to die with dignity' formed the basis of a state duty to treat patients as *they* saw fit, notwithstanding objections from clinicians about whatever the proposed course of treatment was.

Inasmuch as a patient may be especially vulnerable in an intensive care setting (or in any end of life situation), special diligence is required of decision makers. But this is not because of something intrinsic to dying. From a legal perspective, there is nothing special about dying. This chapter is not the place to offer a full analysis of whether dying *should* affect legal freedoms, but we would urge serious consideration of the way the full scheme of the law would be affected before a proposal such as Woods' or Munby J.'s were adopted.[j] The point to make here, however, is that best interests is what the law provides decision makers who are caring for those who lack capacity. Although best interests cannot be boiled down to a single test (or concept),[52] there is a wealth of guidance and principle provided in the case law, the Mental Capacity Act, and the Act's Code of Practice. This principle pervades all medical decision making where consent is unobtainable. Whether you are deciding if you ought to provide a blood transfusion to an unconscious Jehovah's Witness, if you ought to provide antibiotics to treat an infection in a permanently comatose 23-year-old, or if you ought to pump the stomach of a person who has apparently attempted to end their life, you are governed by the constraints and freedoms afforded by best interests. Equally, when you are asked whether it would be lawful to continue medically futile but physically harmless ventilation of a patient in intensive care, in order that the patient's organs may be donated posthumously with a greater chance of success, you are governed by best interests. *Aintree* emphasized that in such cases: […]'the focus is on whether it is in the patient's best interests to give the treatment, rather than on whether it is in his best interests to withhold or withdraw it'[53] (para. 22).

The balancing exercise involved in decision making will necessarily differ from case to case. But the principles run throughout. Thus, it is appropriate to consider how the patient's values would weigh on the decision. That continued ventilation would confer no clinical benefit of itself does not provide compelling reason to withdraw treatment. In the following section, we will demonstrate with three practical examples how the assessments might be made in practice.

---

[j] We would suggest to the interested reader to consider the analysis in Reference 51.

Marrying principle and practice: difficult decisions explored

Consider the following scenarios involving patients in intensive care. Each patient is in a position whereby the medical team justifiably thinks further treatment is clinically futile. Thus, if a decision regarding the patients were to be made purely on medical grounds, withdrawal of treatment would be the indicated course of action.

1. George is 48 years old. He has an organ donor card. He has also told members of his family that he would consent to 'any of my body parts being used if they can be helpful, after I'm dead'.
2. Rubinda is 20 years old. She has not got round to getting an organ donor card because she thought it would be 'tempting fate'. However, her family and friends understand clearly that she viewed posthumous organ donation as a 'strong social duty'.
3. Siobhan is 25 years old. She has never had any profound decision-making capacity, and has never been able to communicate any but the most basic of messages.

Each of the patients could become a donor after death. However, in each case, it would take a few hours for the surgical retrieval team to prepare itself. To optimize the chance of successful retrieval and transplantation, it is suggested that the patients be kept on life support following the futility declaration, until the surgical team is ready. When the team is ready, cardiac arrest would be allowed to happen, and following cardiac death organ retrieval could take place.

Would it be lawful to prolong life support to allow donation to take place in these cases? Let us consider them one by one.

Drawing the line between consent and best interests

In George's case, we are told that he 'would consent' to body parts being retrieved after his death, and that he carries an organ donor card. For many, the act of joining the organ donor register may represent the starkest example of consent to donation, especially given the language that abounds in discussions of these matters, such as 'opt in' and 'opt out'. We ought, however, to acknowledge the complications with this simplification, and the example provided by George gives a helpful opportunity to do so. Consent is a fairly loose term when it applies to matters that happen after we lose capacity: thinking more broadly, one only has to consider the well-rehearsed problems that apply to the applicability or otherwise of advance directives. This chapter is not, and does not pretend to be, a philosophical critique of the alignment of previously expressed wishes by beings whose connectedness to the now extinguished will is corporeal rather than psychological.[k] From a legal perspective, however, we might well question whether the processes involved in obtaining a donor card fulfil the requirements expected for sufficiently informed consent to a procedure. It takes little reflection to notice that a person need hardly—perhaps *can* hardly—be aware of the nature of the processes that might befall his body in order to retrieve his organs, beyond an understanding in the broadest possible terms. Recent jurisprudence, most notably the case of *Montgomery v Lanarkshire Health Board*, has made it established law that, for consent to be 'real', patients must be given information that they would be likely to consider significant and the provision of such information should be by way of dialogue aimed at ensuring the patient understands that information.[56] Mere possession of a donor card, and even a broad expression of will such as that given by George, can hardly be taken as qualifying as informed consent in the sense that medical lawyers have grown to understand it.

This is not a problem. Let us assume—as is almost certainly proper to do—that George has not *consented* to being kept alive for a couple of hours more than would otherwise be the case in order that he might be a better donor. It does not follow that he has *refused* consent. We can still take his expressions as indications of his values in this situation. And his values must bear directly on the decision maker's assessment of what would be in George's best interests. In other words, George is a willing donor. There must, of course, be limits to his willingness. We could not brutalize him, or harm him in some other way, in order to retrieve his organs while hiding behind the pretence of consent. We can, however, recognize that his values regarding donation are altruistic. By losing capacity, he does not suddenly have to be treated as a selfish individual. Both the case law and the Mental Capacity Act require that *his* past and present wishes and feelings, and *his* beliefs and values be considered. The donor card and statement he made may not provide a consent, but they do provide a strong indication that it would be in George's best interests to be kept alive while the organ retrieval team assembled itself. They are evidence that, were

[k] For such critiques, see References 54 and 55.

he told of this situation, he would consent. In the absence of evidence to the contrary, we would suggest that this is an example where best interests would demand that the patient be kept alive, albeit that the principal beneficiaries of the action *appear* not to include him.

Straightforward best interests

Given what we have said about George, there is little of principle to add in the case of Rubinda. From the facts given, we have no reason to believe that there is even an argument that she consents. It seems that she has tried to put her mind away from consideration of this situation. Nevertheless, we once more have an expression of values. However, in Meyers' concept of autonomy (in which she seeks to accommodate both individual and relational autonomy through the concept of the autonomy as self) she cautions that the 'social self' can have a negative impact on the exercise of autonomy where 'the assimilation of culturally transmitted values' may prevent 'critical reflection on the values and desires that shape one's choices'.[57] In light of this and given the reference to Rubinda's view of posthumous organ donation as a 'strong social duty', we might be more extensive in our search for the views of family and others who know the patient, to be sure about the extent of her values. If the evidence is that Rubinda would prefer that she be kept alive in order to optimize the chances of successful donation, were she able to reflect on the situation, it would be perfectly compatible with law that this course of action were pursued. As in the case of George, it would be wrong to infer from lack of consent a refusal of consent. A refusal of consent would be binding. In the absence of consent and refusal, best interests applies. If careful, good faith application of best interests recommends that Rubinda be kept alive, this will be the lawful course of action.

Woods argues that, in the cases of George and Rubinda, we have conflated best interests with respect for patients' wishes, the former being concerned with the patient's welfare and the latter being concerned with patient autonomy. Thus, for Woods, the continuation of treatment to facilitate organ donation is justified on the basis of respect for their wishes, and therefore respect for their right of autonomy, rather than on the basis of their best interests.[58] This argument, however, fails to take account of the requirement to have regard to the patient's past and present wishes *in* the best interests assessment. Thus, respect for a patient's wishes forms part of the assessment of best interests but is not the only factor to be taken into account. For example, Baumann et al. have argued that while NHBOD may be consistent with a patient's pre-viously expressed wishes about posthumous organ donation, continuing treatment in order to facilitate organ donation may be inconsistent with their wishes about their end of life care.[59] It is not our position that the patient's wishes as to organ donation are the only factor to be taken into account in a best interests assessment, rather that they are one factor to be weighed in the balance.

We would emphasize that these scenarios also assume that continued ven-tilation would be physically harmless to the patient. Stammers questions whether it is right to focus solely on distress, and whether we should con-sider other interests such as bodily integrity.[60] In these examples, the patients' bodily integrity has already been invaded but continuing treatment would amount to a continuation of that invasion. As with end of life values, how-ever, we suggest that this is a relevant consideration but one to be weighed in the best interests assessment alongside the patient's desire to be a posthumous organ donor.

Complex best interests

It is only Siobhan's case that raises significant theoretical difficulties. In con-trast with the cases of George and Rubinda, it is possible here to argue that Siobhan has *never* had a sufficiently established scheme of values that she can truly be said to be a willing donor, or that *she* would be benefited by being kept alive. With regard just to posthumous donation, provided 'appropriate con-sent' were given in accordance with the Human Tissue Act 2004, the organ retrieval itself could lawfully be undertaken. However, there is no system of 'appropriate consent' applicable while Siobhan is still alive. Patients who never have had capacity in a relevant sense are much less easily argued to have a will, or value system, that supports donation.

Even so, consideration of the case law may support donation. The reasoning in *Re Y*[61] supported donation, notwithstanding that the patient could not be said to want it. What seemed to be the main benefit—treatment of her sister—was not something the patient would be aware of. Even if we find the reasoning of Connell J to have been excessively stretched, it is possible to see an arguable benefit to Y: she would benefit from a continued relationship with her mother following her sister's treatment. Siobhan will derive no such benefit. Nor can 'family values' come into this. As she will be a posthumous donor, there is no significant chance of her organs being given to family members or others close to her.[l] For a patient who cannot be said ever to have had values that would support donation, it will be very difficult to argue that there will be a significant benefit in being kept alive—even painlessly—for a brief period for the good of others. Some theorists may find this an ugly default position: perhaps the law should not presume that a person's interests are best served by exclusively self-regarding matters.[m] Gillett argues that a relational approach to humans, which he terms the 'solidarity principle', could justify organ donation and measures taken to increase that when a patient's wishes are not known. According to this principle: (1) humans are relational beings who depend on other humans for their well-being; (2) it is rational and good to enhance the lives of other humans; and (3) all humans have an interest in enhancing the lives of others.[63]

While this could be argued to be within the scope of a concept of relational autonomy when a patient's wishes are not known, our argument is not premised on the application of respect for autonomy but on an assessment of the patient's best interests *per* the overall requirements of the Mental Capacity Act, this being the basis for decision making in the case of incapacitated patients. Therefore, we argue that in Siobhan's case, at least from the limited facts given, her best interests require withdrawal of treatment immediately following the futility decision. We accept that there might be an argument if she were from a family or community whose shared values strongly supported donation, but in the absence of such knowledge we would find it difficult to interpret her best interests as including this act of altruism.

Contention for contention's sake?

We do not for a moment underestimate the difficulties for those working in intensive care, whom we appreciate will carry the burden of decision making, and may feel justified in a view that the law—and lawyers—can be of little help in areas of serious moral, political, and social contention. Thus we do not believe that disputes in this area amount simply to contention for the sake of it. However, we are absolutely clear that the principle discussed in this chapter is based on the law as it exists and is to be interpreted. This is supported by the Department of Health's 2009 guidance,[64] which reflects the conclusions drawn here, and we call upon the General Medical Council to revise its current guidance to mirror that of the Department of Health.

---

[l] Directed donation, although permissible for living donors, is not permissible for donation made post-mortem.

[m] See the reasoning in Reference 62.

On timing

One further area of contention, on which the law is unfortunately silent, relates to the timing of NHBOD after cardiac death. The Academy of Medical Royal Colleges' code of practice[65] (p. 12) and the British Transplantation Society's guidelines[66] (p. 11) provide that individuals should be observed for a minimum of five minutes to ensure that cardiac death has occurred, meaning that organ retrieval cannot be commenced before this time has elapsed. Clearly, neither of these amounts to comprehensive *legal* guidance, and a potentially significant issue is raised as situations exist in which the chances of optimizing transplant success would require a shorter period. A paper from the United States discusses three cases where hearts were transplanted from donors who had suffered cardiac death. One was observed for three minutes following the cessation of cardiocirculatory function, the other two for just 75 seconds.[67] If performed in England, it is unclear whether such measures would be lawful or not. On the one hand, it might be argued that if a 'responsible body of medical men skilled in that particular art'[68] (p. 587) supported such practice, the courts would likely find it acceptable, provided there had also been support from family members of the deceased. On the other hand, without a statutory definition of death, and on such a politically and ethically contentious matter, it may be that strict accordance with the guidance is the most sensible approach, notwithstanding that the guidance itself states that it may not apply in every case[69] (p. 6). This, of course, leaves the healthcare practitioners in the invidious position of either facing the risk of falling foul of the law, or of less than optimizing their transplant efforts. The previous edition of this chapter suggested that clarity may be found when the Human Tissue Authority issues guidance on the definition of death. To date, however, it has not done so with its guidance stating that the diagnosis of death is a matter for clinicians[70] (para 59). It is not possible in a chapter with the generality that this has to offer reassurance beyond stating that there is an argument that could be made for the lawfulness of having an observation period of under five minutes following cardiac arrest.

Conclusion

Notwithstanding our sympathy with practitioners working on the front line, we would urge the following two points. First, what we are advocating is not an 'expanded interpretation' of best interests. Best interests, as presented here, is how it exists at law. It is neither expanded nor compounded nor selectively interpreted. Best interests does not under law represent solely an individual patient's clinical needs. The law, both as it developed in the courts, and now as it exists in the Mental Capacity Act, makes this clear. Considering the understanding as 'expanded' will unnerve clinicians for no good reason, and will skew how best interests is rightly understood at law. Second, we caution against an excessive preoccupation with informed consent as it relates to the donor register. As ought to be clear, best interests judgements are necessarily made *absent* consent of the patient, and thus no one would claim that the conditions necessary for lawful consent are (or ought to be) present in the situations considered in this chapter. Nor, as we have demonstrated, should it be assumed that signing on to the donor register serves as informed consent: it is an indication of a willingness to donate given the propitious conditions, which of necessity will be unknown at the time of joining the register. Just as many people are not on the organ donor register, many people have not, for example, made 'living wills', yet practitioners find themselves equipped to make decisions regarding proper treatment of this latter group of patients. It is a cliché, though not necessarily wrong, to observe that doing what is best is not always the same as doing what is easiest. We nevertheless suggest that a proper understanding and application of best interests should pervade *all* decision making for persons who lack capacity. A decision to prolong medically futile ventilation for the reasons considered in this chapter should be subject to no less complete an evaluation than any other decision. Where the patient's values require a modest, harmless prolongation of life for the great potential benefit to others, good practice requires respect for this.

References

1. Bell MDD (2005). Non-heartbeating organ donation: clinical process and fundamental issues. *British Journal of Anaesthesia* **94** (4): 474–478.
2. Gardiner D, Riley B (2007). Non-heart-beating organ donation—solution or a step too far? *Anaesthesia* **62**: 431–433.
3. Baumann A, Audibert G, Layfaye CG, Puybasset L, Mertes PM, Claudot F (2013). Elective non-therapeutic intensive care and the four principles of medical ethics. *Journal of Medical Ethics* **39** (3): 139–142.
4. De Lora P, Blanco AP (2013). Dignifying death and the morality of elective ventilation. *Journal of Medical Ethics* **39** (3): 145–148.
5. Modra L, Hilton A (2015). Ethical issues in organ transplantation. *Anaesthesia and Intensive Care Medicine* **16** (7): 321–323.

6. Coggon J, Brazier M, Murphy P, Price D, Quigley M (2008). Best interests and potential organ donors. *British Medical Journal* **336** (7657): 1346–1347.

7. Coggon J and Murphy P (2011). Ante-mortem issues affecting deceased donation: an ethico-legal perspective, in Farrell A, Price D and Quigley M, *Organ Shortage: Ethics, Law and Pragmatism*, Cambridge University Press, Cambridge.

8. Coggon J (2013). Elective ventilation for organ donation law, policy and public ethics. *Journal of Medical Ethics* **39** (3): 130–134.

9. Coggon J (2016). Mental capacity law, autonomy and best interests: an argument for conceptual and practical clarity. *Medical Law Review* **24** (3): 396–414.

10. Department of Health (2009). Legal Issues Relevant to Non-heart-beating Organ Donation. Available at https://assets.publishing.service.gov.uk/government/uploads/system/uploads/attachment_data/file/138313/dh_109864.pdf (accessed 10 December 2019)

11. General Medical Council (2010). Treatment and Care Towards the End of Life: Good Practice in Decision Making. Available at https://www.gmc-uk.org/-/media/documents/treatment-and-care-towards-the-end-of-life---english-1015_pdf-48902105.pdf (accessed 10 December 2019)

12. Brazier M, Cave E (2016). *Medicine, Patients and the Law*, 6th edn. Manchester University Press, Manchester, pp. 155–6).

13. McGee AJ, White BP (2013). Is providing elective ventilation in the best interests of potential donors? *Journal of Medical Ethics* **39** (3): 135–138.

14. *Learning from Bristol: The Report of the Public Inquiry into Children's Heart Surgery at the Bristol Royal Infirmary 1984–1995* (2001) Cm 5270(1).

15. *The Royal Children's Inquiry Report* (2001) HC 12-11.

16. Bell MDD (2006). Emergency medicine, organ donation and the Human Tissue Act. *Emerg Med J* **23**: 824–827.

17. Department of Health and Social Care (2017). Consultation on Introducing 'Opt-out' Consent for Organ and Tissue Donation in England. Available at https://www.gov.uk/government/consultations/introducing-opt-out-consent-for-organ-and-tissue-donation-in-england/consultation-on-introducing-opt-out-consent-for-organ-and-tissue-donation-in-england (accessed 10 December 2019).

18. Human Tissue Act 2004.

19. Human Transplantation (Wales) Act 2013.

20. *Bolam v. Friern Hospital Management Committee* [1957] 1 WLR 582.

21. *Bolitho v. City and Hackney Health Authority* [1998] AC 232.

22. *In Re T (Adult: Refusal of Treatment)* [1993] Fam 95.

23. *Ms B v An NHS Hospital Trust* [2002] 2 All ER 449.

24. Gray J (1996). *Isaiah Berlin*. Princeton University Press, Princeton, NJ.

25. McGuinness S, Brazier M (2008). Respecting the living means respecting the dead too. *Oxford Journal of Legal Studies* **28** (2): 297–316.

26. Berlin I (1969). Two concepts of liberty, in *Four Essays on Liberty*, Oxford University Press, Oxford.

27. Kong C (2017). *Mental Capacity in Relationship: Decision-making, Dialogue, and Autonomy*, Cambridge University Press, Cambridge.

28. Newdick C, Derrett S (2006). Access, equity and the role of rights in health care. *Health Care Analysis* 14: 157–168.

29. Newdick C (2008). Preserving social citizenship in health care markets: there may be trouble ahead. *McGill Journal of Law and Health* 2: 93–108.

30. Newdick C (2005). *Who Should We Treat? Rights, Rationing and Resources*, 2nd edn. Oxford University Press, Oxford.

31. Syrett K (2007). *Law, Legitimacy and the Rationing of Health Care*. Cambridge University Press, Cambridge.

32. McLean S (2010). *Autonomy, Consent and the Law*, Routledge-Cavendish, Abingdon.

33. *R (On the Application of Oliver Leslie Burke) vs. The General Medical Council* [2005] EWCA Civ 1003.

34. *In Re S (Adult Patient: Sterilisation)* [2001] Fam 15.

35. Coggon and Murphy, Ante-mortem issues affecting deceased donation.

36. *In Re S (Adult Patient: Sterilisation)* [2001] Fam 15.

37. *In Re A (Medical Treatment: Male Sterilisation)* [2000] 1 FCR 193.

38. Coggon J (2008). Best interests, public interest, and the power of the medical profession. *Health Care Analysis* 16 (3): 219–232.

39. *In Re F (Mental Patient: Sterilisation)* [1990] 2 AC 1.

40. *Re Y (Mental Patient: Bone Marrow Donation)* [1997] 2 WLR 556.

41. *Ahsan v University Hospitals Leicester NHS Trust* [2007] PIQR P19.

42. Stammers T (2013). 'Elective' ventilation: an unethical and harmful misnomer? *The New Bioethics* 19 (2): 130–140.

43. Rady MY, Verheijde JL (2013). *Ashan v University Hospitals Leicester NHS Trust* does not legitimize antemortem organ preservation in end-of-life care. *Journal of Medical Ethics* (online). Available at https://jme.bmj.com/content/ahsan-v-university-hospitals-leicester-nhs-trust-does-not-legitimize-antemortem-organ (accessed 10 December 2019).

44. *Aintree University Hospitals NHS Foundation Trust v James* [2013] UKSC 67.

45. *Ms B v An NHS Hospital Trust* [2002] 2 All ER 449.

46. Brazier and Cave, *Medicine, Patients and the Law*.

47. Brazier M (2006). Do no harm—do patients have responsibilities too? *Cambridge Law Journal* 65 (2): 397–422.

48. Woods S (2008). Best interests: puzzles and plausible solutions at the end of life. *Health Care Analysis* 16 (3): 279–287.

49. Woods S (2007). *Death's Dominion: Ethics and the End of Life*. Open University Press, Berkshire.

50. *R (on the application of Burke) v. General Medical Council* [2005] 2 WLR 431.

51. Huxtable R (2008). Whatever you want? Beyond the patient in medical law. *Health Care Analysis* **16** (3): 288–301.

52. Kopelman LM (1997). The best-interests standard as threshold, ideal, and standard of reasonableness. *Journal of Medicine and Philosophy* **22** (3): 271–289.

53. *Aintree University Hospitals NHS Foundation Trust v James* [2013] UKSC 67.

54. McMahan J (2003). *The Ethics of Killing: Problems at the Margins of Life*, Oxford University Press, New York.

55. Wrigley A (2007). Personal identity, autonomy and advance statements. *Journal of Applied Philosophy* **24**(4): 381–396.

56. *Montgomery v. Lanarkshire Health Board* [2015] UKSC 11.

57. Meyers D (2005). Decentralising autonomy: five faces of selfhood', in Christman J, Anderson J, *Autonomy and the Challenges to Liberalism: New Essays*, Cambridge University Press, Cambridge.

58. Woods, S (2011). Book review: law and ethics in intensive care. *Medical Law Review* **19** (3): 495–504.

59. Baumann et al., Elective non-therapeutic intensive.

60. Stammers, 'Elective' Ventilation.

61. *Re Y (Mental Patient: Bone Marrow Donation)* [1997] 2 WLR 556.

62. Harris J, Holm S (2003). Should we presume moral turpitude in our children? – Small children and consent to medical research. *Theoretical Medicine and Bioethics* **24** (2): 121–129.

63. Gillett G (2013). Honouring the donor: in death and in life. *Journal of Medical Ethics* **39** (3): 149–152.

64. Department of Health. Legal Issues Relevant to Non-heart-beating Organ Donation.

65. Academy of Royal Colleges (2008). A Code of Practice for the Diagnosis and Confirmation of Death. Available at http://www.aomrc.org.uk/wp-content/uploads/2016/04/Code_Practice_Confirmation_Diagnosis_Death_1008-4.pdf (accessed 18 December 2019).

66. British Transplantation Society (2004). Guidelines relating to solid organ transplants from non-heart beating donors. Available at https://bts.org.uk/wp-content/uploads/2016/09/NonHeart.pdf (accessed 18 December 2019).

67. Boucek MM, Mashburn C, Dunn SM, et al. (2008). Pediatric heart transplantation after declaration of cardiocirculatory death. *New England Journal of Medicine* **359**: 709–714.

68. *Bolam v. Friern Hospital Management Committee* [1957] 1 WLR 582.

69. Academy of Royal Colleges, A Code of Practice for the Diagnosis and Confirmation of Death.
70. Human Tissue Authority (2017). Code of Practice, Code F: Donation of solid organs and tissue for transplantation. Available at https://www.hta.gov.uk/sites/default/files/files/HTA%20Code%20F.pdf (accessed 18 December 2019).

9

Conflicts of Interest

Neil Soni, the late Andrew Lawson, and Carl Waldmann

Introduction

Of the many definitions of 'conflict of interest', one of the simplest is when an individual, a group of individuals, or an organization has competing interests or loyalties. This may take many guises, including personal versus professional loyalties and interests within or between organizations. Conflicts of interest appear in all walks of life, and indeed may be a normative aspect of society because institutions and individuals may have conflicting obligations that they have to reconcile.

NHS England has a variation on this definition: 'A set of circumstances by which a reasonable person would consider that an individual's ability to apply judgement or act, in the context of delivering, commissioning, or assuring taxpayer funded health and care services is, or could be, impaired or influenced by another interest they hold.' In this version, the focus is quite rightly on the taxpayer.

In the medical profession, conflicts of interest potentially pervade almost all aspects of professional activity and frequently occur in situations where there is supposedly a common interest. If delivery of healthcare is the focus, the broad brush examples might include issues in areas such as service provision and education. They might apply between government and colleges, colleges and individual institutions, institutions and individuals, frequently between cooperating departments and even between individuals in a department. Conflicts of interest are common and are resolved to a greater or lesser degree by reconciliation and compromise.

The two outstanding areas usually highlighted in medicine are those of nepotism in the job market and the interactions between medicine and industry. The former is allegedly of only historic interest due to rigorous, almost draconian, selection procedures. The latter have become in recent years both a recognized problem and the bête noire of the profession.

The relationships between physicians and industry have always been important and are increasingly so in the current economic climate. The positive side of the liaison is that it is increasingly vital for the development and delivery of patient care. It has been responsible for impressive medical advances, new product development and increased research funding, as well as research and assisting in education and its delivery. It is not all positive and it can and has created opportunities for bias, over-consumption, altered perspectives and hence priorities with, on occasion, misuse of public funds. Examples include prescription bias and device and equipment purchase, and publicity round these has led to increasing public awareness and, with it, unfavourable public perception. In the 1980s, the large cash payments and lavish gifts doctors received from drug companies captured public attention and caused concern that physician integrity was falling victim to commercial influences.[1]

That the clash of agendas of the principal players in the healthcare setting may produce a conflict of interest is hardly surprising. On the one hand, industry works principally for shareholders, not patients, and survival or success depends on sales, which in turn depends on doctors who prescribe or use its products. However, on the other hand, the industry has a vested interest in being seen to be a benefactor and to contribute meaningfully to patient wellbeing from which it derives its income. Commercial interest does not necessarily preclude altruism or doing good. However, without profit, companies cannot either fund ongoing research or pay shareholders. The physician's primary role or duty is acting for the benefit of their patients,[2] but they also have a personal agenda to provide an adequate lifestyle for their families, capability for their research programmes, and the ability to facilitate education within their specialties. Patients have a primary aim in maintaining health or life and governments have interests in cost containment, patient welfare, and political survival.

Industry sponsorship of research and guidelines

The forces acting on Western medicine are immense. The demands for medical advances for research output and higher educational standards are only exceeded by the demands by governments to contain healthcare costs and, in particular, overheads on delivering medical care. Research and education overheads are part of the cost structure. In the absence of comprehensive government funding, collaboration between physicians and industry is, and will be, increasingly essential as physicians are end users of the products.

Collaboration entails 'financial linkage' without which the prospect of impressive medical advances, new products for patient care, increased research, and improved education may not be possible. There are already many examples of where this collaboration has translated into improved medical care. Unfortunately, it seems that conflicts of interest are inevitable. The obvious example of drug promotion by medical professionals with financial stakes in the drugs has already eroded public trust in medicine and industry in some quarters.

At the opening of the European Society of Intensive Care Medicine's congress in Berlin in 2007, Dr Professor Jukka Takala made some very pertinent comments on the issue of 'conflicts of interest'. He emphasized that a gap has developed in how research is conducted compared with how it ought to be carried out, focusing on the concerns that occur when industry partners clinicians for the purpose of research. How can we, as physicians, be sure that results are not biased, and therefore be sure that patients do not suffer unnecessarily as a result?[3,4] He pointed out that trials sponsored by pharmaceutical companies were more likely to be published when results had a favourable outcome for their product. This observation has been made by others.[5,6,7,8] If trials, which show no benefit, were similarly publicized, then it would be easier to provide a balanced opinion to readers. He made the following recommendations.

- Practice guidelines should be developed by experts who do not have conflicts. Source data from completed clinical trials should be made available to an external academic coordinating centre for systematic analysis.
- Journals should require statistical confirmation of clinical trial results by external academic sources for all industry-sponsored studies.
- Research institutes should require unrestricted access to the trial database and unlimited rights to publish the results.

The intrinsic risk is that bureaucracy may make such systems unworkable, obstructive, or financially unacceptable. An historical example might have already been seen in both the European and British approaches to streamlining ethics approvals that initially seemed to do the reverse.[9]

In general, the approach to avoidance of conflict of interest by organization has been efficient and effective although costly. The European Medicines Agency requires advisers to declare any interests annually while the National Institute for Health and Care Excellence (NICE) has a policy document on declaring and managing interests in the context of the committee involved. It also details how breaches are to be managed. Following the 2016 publication of the Association of the British Pharmaceutical Society (ABPI) disclosure of interests database, the colleges in the UK have been discussing a proposal to have a register of the interests of clinicians possibly in company with the General Medical Council (GMC). Whether this will happen and whether it will be voluntary or compulsory, and who will run it and pay for it, have not yet been decided.

Conflicts of interest and the 'XIGRIS' story

The issue of conflicts of interest came to the fore in critical care, with activated protein C. *Activated protein C (Xigris)* was the result of 40 years of research and, following the Prowess trial, was heralded as a major advance. It showed a reduced mortality in patients with severe sepsis.[10] As one of the first trials to demonstrate a therapeutic benefit from a new drug in the critically ill with sepsis, it marked the end of a dismal era of repeated failure in clinical trials in this field. It was exciting but expensive. A course of the drug cost £4,500, three times the then daily cost of providing intensive care for a patient. In 2002, at the European Society of Intensive Care Medicine in Barcelona, several hundred participants signed a declaration initiating the Surviving Sepsis Campaign (or SSC).[11] This called on healthcare professionals and their organizations, governments, health agencies, and public to support an initiative to reduce the mortality from sepsis by 25% within five years. Leading international societies came together to develop an evidenced-based set of guidelines (Sepsis Care Initiative, SCI) that could then be rapidly implemented into clinical practice. It was a remarkable achievement but soon the SCI was strongly criticized by some authors.[12] It was suggested that the sponsors of the SSC were too closely aligned with the process. To others, what was contentious was that part of the SSC initially had three sponsors, one of which provided 90% of the financial support.[13] The integrity of the guidelines was questioned on the basis that there was a potential conflict of interest in that it would appear that the guidelines might well confer benefit on the sponsors. The important consideration here was not the nature of the intent but rather the perception of inappropriate influence. If a drug works beyond all reasonable doubt, then marketing and clinical practice should and would have some degree of confluence, but in any situation less ideal than this there will inevitably be suspicion as to the role of that conflict of interest. A crucial point was that this occurred at a time when guidelines were becoming increasingly popular as a means of translating, and by default enforcing, evidence-based medicine to clinical practice. Developing such powerful tools should mandate freedom from any suspicion, real or otherwise, of conflicts of interest.

Guidelines

Developing a guideline combines evidence-based medicine and consensus opinion. It costs money. In the formation of any guideline, there are vested interests, which include a government trying to contain cost while looking for cost-effectiveness, industry trying to market products, enthusiasts trying to drive their own ideas, and patients trying to get a fair and safe deal. Whatever the funding, there will almost always be secondary interests among those involved. The key assumption about guidelines is that, with opinion leaders using an evidence-based approach, quality and hence reliability will be assured.[14,15] There are few studies looking at the quality of guidelines in critical care medicine and they suggest it is low.[16]

Key questions about a proposed guideline might include the following:

- Is this enterprise primarily in the patients' best interests?
- Are those involved, individual clinician, institution, academic body, industry, and government all primarily focused on patient benefit? If not, what are the other areas of interest or conflict?
- Are there specific gains that are not patient-based but which might accrue to any of the interested parties?
- How significant is the issue of cost containment for the state or other funding body in the synthesis of the guideline, and how does it have an impact on the benefit of the guidelines to the individual?

Probably most important is whether a guideline has capacity for change as evidence evolves.

Gifts

Gifts have long been an integral part of human behaviour used to establish or re-affirm relationships. Tied in is the concept of exchange and a temporal element during which the recipient incurs an implied debt—the concept of reciprocity. It is a qualitative phenomenon, not quantitative; the quantitative element being secondary and contextual in nature. The monetary value should be irrelevant.

It is the act of giving and accepting that initiate or continue the relationship. Gift-giving has always been a key part of marketing. In 2012, the pharmaceutical industry spent $89.5 billion on advertising and promotions directed at professionals.[17] The relevant guidelines from the Department of Health in the UK state that staff should 'refuse gifts, benefits, hospitality or sponsorship of any kind which might be seen to compromise their personal judgement or integrity and to avoid seeking to exert influence to obtain preferential consideration'.

The EC Directive 2001/83 Art. 94 stated: 'Where medicinal products are being promoted to persons qualified to prescribe or supply them, no gifts, pecuniary advantages or benefits in kind may be supplied, offered or promised to such persons, unless they are inexpensive and relevant to the practice of medicine or pharmacy.' A conflict of interest is manifested in the form of a gift from the company to a doctor. These can be in many forms and various shapes and sizes: a plastic pen through to travel and accommodation for a congress, sponsorship for attending meetings or an honorarium for talking at a meeting.[18] The gift is supposedly divorced from any obligation but, even if it does not induce an obligation, it surely does engender goodwill.[19] It is a favour-owed reciprocity. The cost is passed on, for example, to the public with higher-priced drugs. This has been described as the 'misuse of public money'.[20,21] Gifts often purchase access but to extrapolate that to purchasing changes in practice may be unfair. Interposed between the two is professional integrity. What price professional integrity among physicians? Maybe it is as suggested by NHS England in a statement that gifts should be declined but 'low cost branded promotional aids may be accepted where they are under the value of a common industry standard of £6 in total, and need not be declared'. There are also guidelines on hospitality.

Even small gifts might compromise clinical judgement.[22,23] A meeting with a pharmaceutical representative might influence practice change where simple company or flattery or both may be the real value of the gift.[24,25] Influence may be more discrete using sponsorship for continuing medical education (CME) with funding for travel or lodging. Incumbent in this is the observation that drug company-sponsored CME has sometimes preferentially highlighted the sponsor's drug.

Patients have views as to the probity of gift giving and taking. In a family practice survey, free meals were more likely to be disapproved of than ballpoint pens but most believed that drug company gifts influenced physician prescribing.[26] As regards treatment choices, informed decisions should be made without external influence. In summary, it is as naïve to think that any gift is dangerous as it is that all gifts are dangerous. The integrity of the physician is of paramount importance.

Innovation and research

Innovation requires time, manpower, and money to bring forward. While ideas may translate into patient benefit eventually, the upfront costs are rarely publicly supported. Hospitals rarely have minimal money for innovation, and competition for charitable funds is fierce. The major source is industry, and is key. Tensions are bound to develop when the immediate goals of the innovator and industry diverge. Compromise is often inevitable and fertile ground for conflict. In pharmaceuticals, the innovator is often industry with a need to test its developments. In a 'win–win' situation, a great drug will bring financial reward to the company and kudos to the clinicians involved. Shareholders will be happy and patients will benefit. Unfortunately, *most developments have marginal or negligible benefits.* As both financial success and clinical research result from positive results there is potential conflict of interest.[27]

Universities now have to be run along business lines and are becoming centres of innovation.[28] This circumvents industry and shareholders, reduces the external conflicts of interest, and returns profits to the university. It also moves the focus of conflict of interest. Academic posts compete for research income and they now need positive results. It also seems that clinicians and institutions need funding to do industry work. Another dilemma. Industry-sponsored research often incentivizes the doctors by incremental payment for each patient recruited. This enhances recruitment. Without an incentive, the trial may fail and the incentive itself is often providing surplus money that can help fund other projects. As both the primary trial and the spin-off research are all for patient benefit, then it would seem ideal. The problems are many. The incentive may be the primary reason for involvement and the secondary projects the real focus jeopardizing the quality of recruitment and hence the results of the primary trial.[29] The driving forces are usually money and kudos. The former is at corporate and personal level but has linkages to assessment exercises and other 'quality measures' of both academic and financial prowess. The latter may be organizational or personal kudos and may be tied to either ambition or job tenure. There is invariable financial linkage.

Education

Education costs money and the sources are limited. Industry needs physicians to know about its products and physicians need education. Pamphlets and mailshots are rarely read. Direct product-focused meetings are not very useful but indirect sponsorship is seen as a way to get information across. It is advertising by association and in some environments a change of practice has been seen.[30]

Industry facilitates education by sponsorship and the quid pro quo is exposure of physicians to their advertising and their product information. Mechanisms that increase the likelihood of the products being discussed, whether by related topics on the programme or using speakers who are likely to speak favourably, will 'enhance' the product's profile. Trojan horse advertising whereby surreptitious use of respected opinion leaders likely to speak favourably about a product is a more effective method, especially at meetings run by respected organizations where the assumption is that such activity cannot happen. Further goodwill can be engendered by generous provision of travel and accommodation. In all these circumstances, professionals with integrity and intelligence are expected to use discretion in how they assimilate information and follow professional guidelines.

Share dealing and consultancy

It has been noted that physicians in research often have early access to information about their own projects or others. Premature disclosure of results or even probable results based on research could constitute 'insider trading', as could share trading using that information. Consultancy advice to investors, either individually or through advisers, could also constitute criminal activity.[31] Clearly there is a fine line between direct and indirect disclosure of information. Ignorance is no defence.

What the medical profession needs

Box 9.1 summarizes what the profession might reasonably expect from industry.

The Achilles heel of medicine is CME. A significant portion of postgraduate education worldwide is industry dependent. It is generally a very positive relationship.

Box 9.1 Industry involvement

Developing new drugs—phenomenally expensive and almost entirely industry driven

New equipment—ideas from medicine and industry but development usually requires industry

Providing information about specific products

Grants for unrelated activities—educational grants

Setting up and running development programmes

Funding research projects

Funding fellows

Assisting running studies

Individual and local education support

Infrastructure and support for international meetings and forum

Assisting with national projects

Supporting national bodies

What does industry need?

Industry needs to develop, test, and sell its products. In each of these endeavours, it needs an effective, unencumbered interface with clinicians. The stringent requirements to bring a product to market through licensing necessitates a close liaison with medicine. A spin-off of these endeavours has been a rising standard of research, but with it increased costs. Paradoxically, this imposes financial restraint on research activity and mandates further industry involvement.

Industry also needs to promote its products. In particular, utility and efficacy need to be promulgated. Studies and publications go so far, but personal opinion and unsolicited recommendation are also useful. In the United Kingdom, NICE is a very useful arbiter but with a limited repertoire. If a product passes their stringent approach, it can circumvent the need for advertising and in some respects is the ultimate advertising tool. NICE will never be a comprehensive service covering all pharmaceuticals and equipment, and industry still needs to get products to market. Doctors and industry must cooperate symbiotically.

Opinion research and industry

In the United States, the level of financial industry involvement is vast, and probably greater than in the UK.[32,33,34] Sales representatives provide an important interface. On occasion, this has led to non-rational prescribing and increased costs of medications.[35] In the United Kingdom, at least in critical care, this is less of an issue. Junior doctors were traditionally perceived to be vulnerable to suggestion.[36,37] More recently, at least in critical care, it would appear that there is less sales activity and it may well be that central purchasers may now be a more worthwhile target. Work experience with doctors, for which the doctor might receive a fee, has been criticized.[38,39,40,41,42,43]

There are legitimate concerns as to industry-sponsored trials. These have increased and author—industry affiliation has also increased.[44] In part, this is due to greater industry engagement and transparency but other influences have been less benign. Examples are historical but instructive. In sponsored studies, selective serotonin reuptake inhibitors (SSRIs) performed better than tricyclics when compared with non-sponsored studies. In 45 of 45 industry-sponsored rheumatology randomized controlled trials (RCTs), the results favoured the sponsor.[45] The odds ratio for an industry-sponsored paper to be favourable was 3.6 (CI 2.6–4.9) and, if it was only assessing RCTs, the number was 4.13 (CI 2.72–6.32).[46,47] Be aware that these were all peer-reviewed papers, usually in highly respected journals. Dubious research techniques should be eliminated. Classic tricks such as testing the trial drug against a placebo, or an ineffective dose, or an altered route of administration should be identified[48]—likewise, recruitment selectivity, drop-out rates, late exclusions or inclusions, or altering the outcome measures.[49] In a survey of review articles, details of techniques used in trials were rarely reported, and neither were potential conflicts of interest.[50] Journals try and enforce codes of practice in publication and insist on listing conflicts of interest, as do meetings. Reviewers try to look for deviation from acceptable practice, and most researchers do adhere to what they consider good practice. It is clearly not enough but how this can be improved without even more draconian regulations is unclear.

UK codes and regulation

In reality, there is a highly successful and symbiotic relationship between medicine and industry. In the United Kingdom, the pharmaceutical industry has developed robust guidelines acknowledging both the need to foster relationships and defining clear rules of engagement, including a disclosure database. There are specific guidelines for industry involvement in publication. The Royal College of Physicians has a code of conduct that is representative of the central thrust of most other codes.[51]

Speakers cannot be chosen solely by the company and sponsorship must be openly declared. Hospitality for speakers is acceptable but should be commensurate with what they themselves or their employer might provide. Any honoraria and expenses should be handled through an independent scientific body. Support to attend meetings, whether registration, travel, or accommodation, should again be acceptable but should not exceed that which the person or their employer might reasonably supply. The attendance at the meeting should be in the interests of the service, be free of commercial pressure, and not be touristic in nature. There are clear guidelines on accompanying persons. Local meetings should be educational with only modest support, and again clear guidelines exist. Grant scholarships are acceptable but the funds must rest with the institution.

The guidelines regarding research are more complex. Financial matters should bypass the involved clinicians and there should be no financial interest for either clinicians or patients. Indemnity must be provided. With regards to gag clauses, there should be free access to data, independent analysis, and no restraint on publication.[14] It is imperative that academic institutions adopt and uniformly enforce these standards despite potential short-term financial losses. Delays for patent application are approved but should be short. There must be clear declarations of interest. The rules of engagement for clinicians working with or advising companies are clearly stated. Indeed, this document should be mandatory reading for all doctors.

Industry has specific and far-reaching guidelines regarding its interface with the medical profession. In the United Kingdom, the ABPI is very active and has an impressive Code of Practice (2016), which is currently being updated. Industry is well informed of the rules by which doctors must operate, but there is a curious lack of information for doctors about the rules under which industry operates.

Conclusions

Despite the bad press, significant conflicts of interest with potentially damaging outcomes are relatively rare but highly publicized when detected. Medicine and industry need to be symbiotic and government should facilitate such a relationship. Strong regulatory authorities need to establish clear and obvious behaviour boundaries to inhibit abuse without being so draconian as to make cooperation impossible. A pragmatic approach requires the involvement of those active in research engaging with industry rather than disengaged bureaucrats. In any situation where the interests of multiple institutions and individuals coalesce, there are necessarily bound to be conflicts. In healthcare, it is the interests of the patients that are paramount. There have been problems but, given the size of the industry and the complexity of modern healthcare, the incidence of patient harm following on conflicts of interest is probably low. Excessive and over-intrusive regulation may produce an example of the law of unintended consequences whereby patients suffer through stifling of innovation. Recognizing the problem is in itself a form of solution.

Some useful addresses

- Code of Practice for the Pharmaceutical Industry, 2016: https://www.pmcpa.org.uk (accessed 15 December 2019).
- Managing Conflicts of Interest in the NHS, 2017, NHS England: https://www.england.nhs.uk (accessed 15 December 2019).
- EFPIA CODE ON THE PROMOTION OF PRESCRIPTION-ONLY MEDICINES TO, AND INTERACTIONS WITH, HEALTHCARE PROFESSIONALS. EFPIA HCP code (2014): https://www.efpia.eu/media/24302/3a_efpia-hcp-code-2014.pdf (accessed 29 December 2019); Professional Standards for Public Health 2014: https://www.rpharms.com/recognition/setting-professional-standards/professional-standards-for-public-health (accessed 15 December 2019).
- ISPOR Code of Ethics 2017. International Society for Pharmacoeconomics and Outcomes Research: https://www.ispor.org/docs/default-source/resources/codeofethics-guideline.pdf?sfvrsn=bc601080_2 (accessed 15 December 2019).
- Medicines adherence: involving patients in decisions about prescribed medicines and supporting adherence—NICE guideline. 2009. https://nice.org.uk/guidance/cg76 (accessed 15 December 2019). Royal College of Physicians: https://www.rcplondon.ac.uk (accessed 15 December 2019).
- Research Ethics Committee—Standard Operating Procedure, 2018: https://www.hra.nhs.uk/about-us/committees-and-services/res-and-recs/research-ethics-committee-standard-operating-procedures (accessed 15 December 2019).

- Disclosure UK: https://www.abpi.org.uk/our-ethics/disclosure-uk/about-disclosure-uk (accessed 15 December 2019).
- NICE Declarations of interest policy: http://gmmmg.nhs.uk/docs/guidance/GMMMG%20Declarations%20of%20interest%20policy_.pdf (accessed 15 December 2019).

References

1. Katz D, Caplan AL, Merz JF (2003). All gifts large and small: toward an understanding of the ethics of pharmaceutical industry gift-giving. *Am J Bioeth*. **3** (3): 39–46.
2. Gale EA (2003). Between two cultures: the expert clinician and the pharmaceutical industry. *Clin Med*. **3** (6): 538–541.
3. Lexchin J, Bero LA, Djulbegovic B, Clark O (2003). Pharmaceutical industry sponsorship and research outcome and quality: systematic review. *BMJ*. **326** (7400): 1167–1170.
4. Kjaergard LL, Als-Nielsen B (2002). Association between competing interests and authors' conclusions: epidemiological study of randomized clinical trials published in the BMJ. *BMJ*. **325** (7358): 249.
5. Als-Nielsen B, Chen W, Gluud C, Kjaergard LL (2003). Association of funding and conclusions in randomized drug trials: a reflection of treatment effect or adverse Events? *J Am Med Assoc*. **290** (7): 921–928.
6. Brown A, Kraft D, Schmitz SM, Sharpless V, Martin C, Shah R, et al. (2006). Association of industry sponsorship to published outcomes in gastrointestinal clinical research. *Clin Gastroenterol Hepatol*. **4** (12): 1445–1451.
7. Felson DT, Glantz L (2004). A surplus of positive trials: weighing biases and reconsidering equipoise. *Arthritis Research & Therapy*. **6** (3): 117–119.
8. Hartmann M, Knoth H, Schulz D, Knoth S (2003). Industry-sponsored economic studies in oncology vs studies sponsored by nonprofit organisations. *Br J Cancer*. **89** (8): 1405–1408.
9. Stewart PM, Stears A, Tomlinson JW, Brown MJ (2008). Regulation—the real threat to clinical research. *BMJ*. **337**: a1732.
10. Bernard GR, Vincent JL, Laterre PF, LaRosa SP, Dhainaut JF, Lopez-Rodriguez A, et al. (2001). Efficacy and safety of recombinant human activated protein C for severe sepsis. *N Engl J Med*. **344** (10): 699–709.
11. Dellinger RP, Carlet JM, Masur H, Gerlach H, Calandra T, Cohen J, et al. (2004). Surviving Sepsis Campaign guidelines for management of severe sepsis and septic shock. *Intensive Care Med*. **30** (4): 536–555.

12. Eichacker PQ, Natanson C, Danner RL (2006). Surviving sepsis—practice guidelines, marketing campaigns, and Eli Lilly. *N Engl J Med.* **355** (16): 1640–1642.

13. Dellinger et al., Surviving Sepsis Campaign.

14. Penston J (2007). Patients' preferences shed light on the murky world of guideline-based medicine. *J Eval Clin Pract.* **13** (1): 154–159.

15. Rashidian A, Eccles MP, Russell I (2008). Falling on stony ground? A qualitative study of implementation of clinical guidelines' prescribing recommendations in primary care. *Health Policy.* **85** (2): 148–161.

16. Sinuff T, Patel RV, Adhikari NK, Meade MO, Schunemann HJ, Cook DJ (2008). Quality of professional society guidelines and consensus conference statements in critical care. *Crit Care Med.* **36** (4): 1049–1058.

17. Fickweiler F, Fickweiler W, Urbach E (2017). Interactions between physicians and the pharmaceutical industry generally and sales representatives specifically and their association with physicians' attitudes and prescribing habits: a systematic review. *BMJ Open,* **7** (9): e016408.

18. Desmet C (2003). Pharmaceutical firms' generosity and physicians: legal aspects in Belgium. *Med Law.* **22** (3): 473–487.

19. Sandberg WS, Carlos R, Sandberg EH, Roizen MF (1997). The effect of educational gifts from pharmaceutical firms on medical students' recall of company names or products. *Acad Med.* **72** (10): 916–918.

20. DeMaria AN (2007). Your soul for a pen? *J Am Coll Cardiol.* **49** (11): 1220–1222.

21. Iserson KV, Cerfolio RJ, Sade RM (2007). Politely refuse the pen and note pad: gifts from industry to physicians harm patients. *Ann Thorac Surg.* **84** (4): 1077–1084.

22. Washlick JR, Welch SS (2008). Physician–vendor marketing and financial relationships under attack. *J Health Life Sci Law.* **2** (1): 151, 153–228.

23. Coyle SL (2002). Physician–industry relations. Part 2: organizational issues. *Ann Intern Med.* **136** (5): 403–406.

24. Blumenthal D, Causino N, Campbell E, Louis KS (1996). Relationships between academic institutions and industry in the life sciences—an industry survey. *N Engl J Med.* **334** (6): 368–373.

25. Wazana A (2000). Gifts to physicians from the pharmaceutical industry. *JAMA.* **283** (20): 2655–2658.

26. Fadlallah R, Nas H, Naamani D et al. (2016). Knowledge, beliefs and attitudes of patients and the general public towards the interactions of physicians with the pharmaceutical and the device industry: a systematic review. *PLos One.* **11** (8): e0160540.

27. Friedberg M, Saffran B, Stinson TJ, Nelson W, Bennett CL (1999). Evaluation of conflict of interest in economic analyses of new drugs used in oncology. *JAMA.* **282** (15): 1453–1457.

28. Evans GR, Packham DE (2003). Ethical issues at the university-industry interface: a way forward? *Sci Eng Ethics.* **9** (1): 3–16.

29. Ashar BH, Miller RG, Getz KJ, Powe NR (2004). Prevalence and determinants of physician participation in conducting pharmaceutical-sponsored clinical trials and lectures. *J Gen Intern Med.* **19** (11): 1140–1145.

30. Blumenthal D, Campbell EG, Causino N, Louis KS (1996). Participation of life-science faculty in research relationships with industry. *N Engl J Med.* **335** (23): 1734–1749.

31. Freestone DS, Mitchell H (1993). Inappropriate publication of trial results and potential for allegations of illegal share dealing. *BMJ.* **306** (6885): 1112–1114.

32. Blumenthal et al., Participation of life-science faculty.

33. Campbell EG, Weissman JS, Ehringhaus S, Rao SR, Moy B, Feibelmann S, et al. (2007). Institutional academic industry relationships. *JAMA.* **298** (15): 1779–1786.

34. Campbell EG, Louis KS, Blumenthal D (1998). Looking a gift horse in the mouth: corporate gifts supporting life sciences research. *JAMA.* **279** (13): 995–999.

35. Whiteway DE (2001). Physicians and the pharmaceutical industry: a growing embarrassment and liability. *WMJ.* **100** (9): 39–44, 57.

36. Lichstein PR, Turner RC, O'Brien K (1992). Impact of pharmaceutical company representatives on internal medicine residency programs. A survey of residency program directors. *Arch Intern Med.* **152** (5): 1009–1013.

37. Wazana A (2000). Physicians and the pharmaceutical industry: is a gift ever just a gift? *JAMA.* **283** (3): 373–380.

38. Wall LL, Brown D (2002). Pharmaceutical sales representatives and the doctor/patient relationship. *Obstet Gynecol.* **100** (3): 594–599.

39. Drack G, Kuhn HP, Haller U (2003). Is continuing medical education under suspicion of corruption? Contribution to the discussion by the committee for quality preservation of the swiss society of gynaecology and obstetrics. [German]. *Gynakologisch Geburtshilfliche Rundschau.* **43** (2): 111–117.

40. Bero LA, Galbraith A, Rennie D (1992). The publication of sponsored symposiums in medical journals. *N Engl J Med.* **327** (16): 1135–1140.

41. Carney SL, Nair KR, Sales MA, Walsh J (2001). Pharmaceutical industry-sponsored meetings: good value or just a free meal? *Intern. Med. J.* **31** (8): 488–491.

42. Bennett J, Collins J (2002). The relationship between physicians and the biomedical industries: advice from the Royal College of Physicians. *Clin Med.* **2** (4): 320–322.

43. Wilson FS (2003). Continuing medical education: ethical collaboration between sponsor and industry. *Clinical Orthopaed Related Res Issue.* **412**: 33–37.

44. Buchkowsky SS, Jewesson PJ (2004). Industry sponsorship and authorship of clinical trials over 20 years. *Ann Pharmacother.* **38** (4): 579–585.

45. Fries JF, Krishnan E (2004). Equipoise, design bias, and randomized con-
    trolled trials: the elusive ethics of new drug development. *Arthritis Res Ther.* **6**
    (3): R250–R255.

46. Bekelman JE, Li Y, Gross CP (2003). Scope and impact of financial conflicts of
    interest in biomedical research: a systematic review. *JAMA.* **289** (4): 454–465.

47. Kjaergard LL, Nikolova D, Gluud C (1999). Randomized clinical trials in
    hepatology: predictors of quality. *Hepatology.* **30** (5): 1134–1138.

48. Ibid.

49. Peloso PM, Riley ML (1998). Controlled clinical trials and clinical patient-
    care: sometimes in conflict. *Ann R Coll Physicians Surg Can.* **31** (8): 372–374.

50. Roundtree AK, Kallen MA, Lopez-Olivo MA, Kimmel B, Skidmore B, Ortiz Z,
    et al. (2009). Poor reporting of search strategy and conflict of interest in over 250
    narrative and systematic reviews of two biologic agents in arthritis: a systematic
    review. *J Clin Epidemiol.* **62** (2): 128–137.

51. Bennett et al., The relationship between physicians and the biomedical industries.

10

Social Media in Intensive Care

Rosaleen Baruah

Introduction

There is no universally accepted definition of 'social media'. This is perhaps because social media itself is a constantly evolving phenomenon. All forms of social media share certain characteristics that can be used to provide a working definition. Social media providers use websites and web-based internet applications ('apps') that allow users to generate and share content within the website or app. This is known as a 'social media platform'. A platform allows content—written material, pictures, and video—to be displayed in such a way as to enable and encourage interaction with other users. Social media providers optimize their websites and applications to maximize their functionality on mobile devices such as smartphones and tablets, which allows users to update their content wherever they may be located. Platforms may be largely collaborative in nature, such as Wikipedia or YouTube, based around active interaction, such as Facebook or LinkedIn, blog sites such as 'Life in the Fast Lane' or 'EMCrit', or a micro-blogging service such as Twitter. Discussion fora such as those provided by the website doctors.net.uk, allow discussion between medical professionals on a secure platform intended for use only by verified registered medical practitioners.

By building a community of fellow users in a social media network, a user can produce a self-generated, constantly modified internet space full of content that is relevant to them and their fellow users.[1] Algorithms generated by the social media platform designers ensure that the content viewed by the user, including advertisements, is tailored to the user's perceived interests. On joining a network, a user is prompted to create a 'profile', which includes personal demographic details and personal and professional interests. Depending on the platform being used, users can then share updates, links, photographs, and video clips.

The most popular social media platforms (Facebook, Twitter, Instagram) allow users to label content using 'hashtags'. Labelling content with a hashtag allows it to be found more easily using the search function of the application. For example, if an educational update on Twitter (a 'tweet') was labelled with the hashtag '#FOAMEd', (a popular hashtag used to identify content that provides free, open access medical education), any user searching for this content would be able to find this tweet by searching for this hashtag. Multiple hashtags can be attached to any one piece of content, maximizing its exposure. A piece of content on social media that receives widespread exposure (often involving millions of 'shares' or views) is said to have 'gone viral'. A topic that is being discussed widely on social media is described as a 'trending' topic.

Popular social media platforms

The use of social media platforms has increased steadily since their development in the early 2000s. Usage of social media platforms is now part of everyday life for a sizable proportion of the world's population. Facebook estimated it had 2.45 billion monthly active users in the third quarter of 2019.[2] Twitter, in the same time period, was estimated to have 336 million monthly active users.[3] A 2016 study[4] found that blogs were the most popular form of social media used by doctors in the USA for professional purposes, followed by Twitter and Facebook. A 2017 OFCOM report found that the majority of adult social media users had multiple accounts with different platforms, with only 32% using one platform only.[5] A survey of social media use for professional reasons in the USA revealed that medical students had the highest rate of social media use at 93.5% and approximately 40% of practising physicians regularly used social media in their professional lives.[6]

Social media and harassment

In 2017 and 2018, two cases in United Kingdom (UK) paediatric intensive care units (ICUs) demonstrated the use of social media in rapidly spreading the story of a patient and family to an international audience, and its use in attempting to change the proposed treatment plan for the patient by applying pressure through social media platforms. In 2017, the case of Charlie Gard, a young boy with severe brain damage secondary to mitochondrial disease, gained much international coverage via social media, using the Facebook group 'Charlie's Army' and the hashtag #charliesarmy. The Pope and the US President tweeted their support for Charlie's family, arguing against withdrawal of life-sustaining treatment.[7] Francis J, in his judgment confirming his initial declaration that withdrawal of ventilation and initiation of palliative care were in Charlie's best interests, commented that 'the world of social media doubtless has very many benefits but one of its pitfalls … is that when cases such as this go viral, the watching world feels entitled to express opinions, whether or not they are evidence-based'.[8] The following year, the case of Alfie Evans, a young child with severe brain damage of unknown aetiology gained exposure through social media. A post from 'Alfie's Army', a Facebook group dedicated to publicizing the case, was seen by a 'pro-life' activist affiliated to a Christian pressure group known as the 'Christian Legal Centre',[9] which then began acting on behalf of Alfie Evans' parents in objecting to the hospital's efforts to obtain a declaration permitting withdrawal of life-sustaining treatment. Using the Alfie's Army Facebook group and the hashtag #alfiesarmy on Twitter, support for the Evans' family was raised internationally, including again from the Pope and the US President. Social media was used to organize large and vocal protests at the hospital, including generating plans to 'storm' the hospital and disrupt its clinical work by setting off fire alarms.[10] Social media was also used to deliver 'a barrage of highly abusive and threatening language and behaviour' directed at staff working in the hospital.[11]

There is evidence that people who engage in online harassment may be encouraged to do so by their online environments, and that individuals who in all other respects are law-abiding citizens may participate in this form of antisocial behaviour. Users of social media may choose to remain anonymous or use a pseudonym, and this anonymity may promote a sense of de-individualization, social normalization of aberrant behaviour, and lack of individual accountability.[12] This in turn may facilitate online communications that may be far more aggressive and, in some cases, threatening and violent, than the given individual would ever participate in in face-to-face situations. Being a member of a social media group or thread, in which the overall tone of messages is aggressive and threatening, may lower the threshold of all participants for engaging in verbally aggressive online behaviour.[13] This phenomenon was observed in the cases of Charlie Gard and Alfie Evans. In the case of Alfie Evans, discussions in the 'Alfie's Army' Facebook group initially centred around sharing news of, and support for, Alfie and his family, before escalating to plans to storm the hospital and disrupt clinical services.

Online harassment is a frequent occurrence for users of social media. Registered medical practitioners, who are encouraged by the General Medical Council (GMC) to identify themselves by their full names if they identify as doctors on social media, can easily be found on social media by those with the intent to harass them. The 2017 OFCOM report on adult media use found that 14% of those surveyed had been exposed to 'nasty or aggressive' comments about them on social media.[14] The Pew Center, a US-based organization that maps social trends, found a higher incidence of abusive behaviour online, with 27% of respondents reporting being subject to offensive name-calling and 22% to purposeful embarrassment. More severe behaviours, such as sustained harassment, online stalking, and sexual harassment were considerably rarer.[15]

Online harassment can take several forms and fall anywhere along a spectrum ranging from unpleasant name calling and antagonistic comments to wishing unpleasant events to happen to the subject of abuse, to directs threats of serious physical and sexual assault, to murder. Such threats can occur directly, by having messages sent straight to users via a social media platform, or indirectly as was the case for hospital staff in the Evans case, where threats were made on the pages dedicated to advocating for Alfie Evans and his family. 'Trolling' is a form of abuse that is particular to social media and can be defined as 'seeking satisfaction in provoking negative emotions in others'[16] by posting deliberately oppositional, provoking material that may not in itself appear abusive in nature. Social media platform providers have their own 'house rules' that everyone using the site is expected to adhere to. Users who find themselves the target of abusive or threatening contact via a social media platform may alert the platform directly, and users who engage in such behaviour may have their access to the platform suspended or permanently disabled. Given that platforms do not require verification of a user's identity to set up an account, there is nothing to stop an online harasser opening a new account to continue their harassment. The British Medical Association, in its guide, 'Social media—practical guidance and best practice,'[17] provides guidance for dealing with challenging social media encounters. In the event of engaging in communications that may have become heated, they recommend either withdrawing from the interaction or, if appropriate, 'unfollowing' or blocking the user. Persistent harassment should be dealt with in line with the policy of each individual platform.

Serious threats delivered via social media may constitute a criminal offence, and in 2016 the Crown Prosecution Service published guidance detailing increased powers for prosecuting those who engage in online harassment and trolling.[18] The types of offence dealt with fall under three categories; communications that may constitute threats of violence to the person or damage to property; communications that specifically target an individual or individuals and which may constitute harassment, stalking, or controlling behaviour; or communications that may amount to a breach of a court order or a statutory prohibition. Table 10.1 details individual threats and the Acts that they would fall under:

Table 10.1 Criminal communication via social media and corresponding legislation

Threat to kill	Offences Against the Person Act 1861
Threat of violence to the person	Protection from Harassment Act 1977
	Malicious Communications Act 1988
	Communications Act 2003
Hostility based on race or religion	Crime and Disorder Act 1998
Hostility based on sexual orientation	Public Order Act 1986
False or offensive social media profile	Public Order Act 1986
Libellous statements	Defamation Act 2013

It is possible that an individual may be charged under more than one of the Acts depending on the nature of the offence.

Guidelines for use of social media by healthcare professionals in the United Kingdom

The success of social media relies on developing a culture where openness and sharing are the norm. This is at odds with traditional medical ethical values such as confidentiality and privacy. Social media can be used for both social and professional purposes, which can lead to an unhelpful blurring of lines between personal and professional roles. For example, a photograph shared on Twitter of a group of healthcare professionals attending a conference dinner and clearly consuming alcohol may be viewed negatively by members of the general public, despite such events being entirely commonplace at medical meetings and the consumption of alcohol at such evenings a standard behaviour that would not otherwise attract comment or action from any regulatory body. Users of social media may feel a sense of detachment from the content they post and may behave online in a way they would not behave in real life.[19] There is also evidence suggesting that users will, when questioned, voice concerns over their privacy online, but when actually using social media they may demonstrate much less concern over sharing large amounts of personal information and opinion—the so-called 'privacy paradox.'[20] Posts on social media have the potential to spread globally in a very short period of time. Healthcare professionals using social media therefore need to be aware of their professional responsibilities when using social media platforms.

Healthcare professionals who use social media inappropriately face censure by their regulatory bodies.[21,22] The GMC has produced guidelines for the use of social media for doctors.[23] The guidance states clearly that the standards expected of doctors' online communication via social media are the same as those expected when communicating via more traditional methods, or face to face. Persistent or serious failure to adhere to the principles of the guidance will put a practitioner's professional registration at risk.

The guidance from the GMC falls under the broad categories of privacy, boundaries, confidentiality, respect for colleagues, conflicts of interest, and anonymity. The spirit of the guidance is in keeping with *Good Medical Practice*[24] and *Confidentiality: good practice in handling patient information*.[25]

Notably, the guidance states that 'if you identify yourself as a doctor in publicly accessible social media, you should also identify yourself by name'.[26] The justification given for this is that anyone representing themselves as a doctor on social media is likely 'to be taken on trust [by members of the public] and may reasonably be taken to represent the views of the profession more widely'.[27] This was seen as a controversial statement by the profession when the guidelines were first released and some doctors voiced concerns that, by limiting the ability of medical practitioners to post anonymously online, their rights under articles 8 and 10 of the Human Rights Act 1998, which guarantees a right to a private life and freedom of speech, would be infringed.[28] An online e-petition demanding retraction of the guideline and preservation of doctors' rights to post anonymously online was organized by UK doctors and sent to the Department of Health after garnering over 4,000 signatures. Following this, the GMC took the step of issuing a statement of clarification on its Facebook page.[29] This stated that the guidance to identify oneself as a doctor applied to social media activity that dealt with medical issues, or espoused opinions on medical matters. The guidance only restricts doctors' rights to post online if doing so would breach patient confidentiality, or when online activity involves bullying, harassing, or making malicious comments about a colleague online, all of which are in alignment with the principles of *Good Medical Practice*, the core guidance regulating doctors' performance in the UK. The guidance uses the term 'you should' rather than 'you must', which allows doctors to exercise professional judgement when posting online, and therefore was not viewed by the GMC as infringing the online free speech of the medical profession.

The Nursing and Midwifery Council (NMC), the body responsible for setting standards of conduct for nurses and midwives in the UK, has produced guidance on using social media responsibly.[30] This guidance integrates the principles of *The Code: professional standards of practice and behaviour for nurses and midwives*.[31] The guide states that registration is at risk if an individual's behaviour on social media is unprofessional or unlawful. These behaviours include: sharing confidential information inappropriately; posting pictures of patients and people receiving care without their consent; posting inappropriate comments about patients; bullying, intimidating, or exploiting people; building or pursuing relationships with patients; stealing personal information or using someone else's identity; encouraging violence or self-harm; and inciting hatred or discrimination.[32] The NMC's document is somewhat more comprehensive in its guidance, but it does not specifically impose a duty on its registrants to identify themselves by name on social media if they identify themselves as a registered nurse.

Benefits of social media use by healthcare professionals in critical care

There are clear disadvantages to use of social media, if used inappropriately. Responsible use of social media platforms can, however, be a force for good. National professional associations such as the UK Faculty of Intensive Care Medicine, Intensive Care Society and British Association of Critical Care Nurses all have Twitter accounts with a combined following of 21,000 account holders, allowing free publicity of these groups' events and initiatives. Public health campaigns supporting sepsis awareness and organ donation, for example, now provide specific resources to encourage sharing of awareness on social media by healthcare professionals and members of the public.[33,34] The #hellomynameis campaign is an excellent example of the use of social media, in this case mainly Twitter, to spread awareness of the importance of healthcare professionals introducing themselves clearly, by name, to patients and their families.[35]

Benefits of active social media use by intensive care professionals include keeping up with current literature, being exposed to ideas they otherwise may not gain exposure to, engaging in discussions with colleagues, opening up career or research opportunities, and providing a means of expressing personal opinions. Conversely, barriers to social media use include lack of familiarity with the platforms, fears of negative responses, being accused of unprofessional behavior, or breaching patient confidentiality.[36,37]

Social media and its use in medical education

Social media is increasingly used as a medium for medical education, and a vast amount of medical educational content is freely available on platforms. For example, a search on the video-sharing platform YouTube for 'central line insertion' generates 236,000 results.[38]

Social media, and in particular Twitter, has become a key method of disseminating information from medical conferences and meetings.[39] A meeting will advertise in advance a hashtag that users can include in their social media posts to allow other users to search for content about the meeting—for example, #ICSSOA2019 for the Intensive Care Society 2019 State of the Art Meeting. Content from a meeting can thus be shared around the world in real time, facilitating dissemination of information and professional networking.

As it is widely available worldwide, the internet has allowed for a democratization of the production of medical education resources. This democratization allows greater participation by members of the profession who perhaps would not have previously been involved in producing mass market education resources, but it also brings with it ethical concerns regarding patient confidentiality and quality of the materials produced and distributed.

'Crowdsourcing' refers to online material that has been authored by multiple voluntary online contributors. The database or website produced as a result of this crowdsourced effort is known as a 'wiki' (Hawaiian for 'quick', referring to the relative speed of establishing, and editing, information within the wiki). There are a number of crowdsourced medical wikis online, such as WikiEM and Radiopedia, in addition to Wikipedia, the largest wiki in existence. A key principle of a wiki is that is openly editable, meaning any user can modify content on the platform. Being openly editable allows wikis to remain completely up to date provided users have made appropriate edits. There is also an inherent risk that the openly editable nature of the wiki model allows misinformation to be presented to a wide audience online.

The quality and accuracy of medical educational material contained within wikis or disseminated via other social media sites can be challenging to verify. The Health on the Net Foundation is an organization that serves as a quality marker for health-related resources on the internet and was founded in 1996 with the aim 'to promote the deployment of useful and reliable health information online and to enable its appropriate and efficient use.'[40] A medical site that has signed up to its eight HONCode principles agrees to regular independent audit of quality of content, which gives users some assurance as to the quality of information contained within the website. The HONCode, however, only mandates disclosure of the credentials of the moderators of a site or wiki, not the credentials of each individual contributor. A study examining the quality of medical wikis found only 10 out of the 25 studied required users' credentials to gain editing rights.[41] While some organizations and journals have YouTube channels and Twitter accounts that are verified (this requires the account holder to provide the social media platform with evidence to verify their identity), the majority of social media #FOAMEd tweets do not carry such a guarantee of authenticity.

The UK GMC makes it clear that doctors have an obligation to keep their professional knowledge and skills up to date[42] and the bite-sized nature of social media-based education can seem a very effective way of delivering this. It is essential, however, that sources of such education are from sites and authors whose identities and affiliations can be verified as being up to date and reliable. There is no obligation for authors of free open access medical education or wiki contributors to declare potential conflicts of interest, which may include financial conflicts of interest, when contributing to social media-based medical education. The UK GMC places an obligation on registered medical practitioners to declare any such conflicts of interest. The onus is on the practitioner to use professional judgement to identify when such a conflict of interests may arise, and to avoid these whenever possible.[43] For example, a doctor who acts as a paid consultant to a company producing airway devices should avoid promoting the company's devices in a Twitter discussion on airway management, unless they make clear their affiliation with the device manufacturer.

Social media and families on the intensive care unit

Social media is frequently used by families whose loved ones are patients in an ICU. The social media feeds generated by these families may contain pictures and video clips of the patient, written updates of the patient's condition, and accounts of discussions with members of the treating team. Privacy settings of social media feeds can ensure that this material is only shared with close family and friends, but, if desired, families can allow photos, videos, and status updates to be seen by any platform account holder worldwide. Social media may also be used by patients who are discharged from the ICU as a means of communicating with fellow survivors. These groups can be hosted by institutions,[44] may be moderated by hospital staff, or may be independent groups on platforms such as Facebook.[45]

Social media feeds by families of patients on an ICU can generate considerable attention within social media and traditional media. Here we discuss the ethical aspects of the sharing of clinical details and images of patients who have not provided explicit consent for this material to be shared, by virtue of age or loss of decision-making capacity.

There have been high-profile cases in the UK involving widespread use of social media in ICUs, such as the cases of Charlie Gard and Alife Evans. These cases, discussed earlier under 'Social media and harassment', involved conflict between family and doctors in determining whether life-sustaining treatment should continue. There are many other children and adults whose admissions to an ICU are documented by their families on social media, with the intention of updating family and friends and wider groups of supporters, and of raising awareness of serious childhood conditions.[46] Adults who have been admitted to an ICU can have their admission documented by their families and friends, or have their own social media accounts used by their families to allow photographs, videos, and status updates of their progress to be added to their feed.

Adults admitted to an ICU are very likely to have lost some, if not all, decision-making capacity and are not in a position to give permission to their family to have their ICU admission documented on social media. Children are not permitted to open their own accounts on the majority of social media platforms until they have reached the age of 13, and some platforms such as Twitter allow access to 13–18-year-olds only under supervision of a parent or legal guardian,[47] and so children in this age group will only be exposed on social media via the accounts of others.

The nature of critical illness, and the physical burden of ICU care, render patients vulnerable to psychological distress during and after their admission, and it is arguable that having details, including visual images, of their stay in the ICU distributed over social media may compound this. There is some evidence that children may be adversely affected by their images and details of their lives being shared by their parents on social media, so-called 'sharenting'[48] with negative aspects including the risk of sharing potentially embarrassing personal information that may later follow the child into adulthood as part of the child's 'digital footprint'. Article 16 of the United Nations Convention on the Rights of the Child (UNCRC), which came into force in the UK in 1992, places an obligation on countries that have ratified it to 'protect the child's private, family and home life, including protecting children from unlawful attacks that harm their reputation'.[49] Article 8 of the European Convention on Human Rights (ECHR) and enshrines the right to respect for private and family life. Distributing material on social media, without explicit permission, which documents the ICU admission of a patient who has no capacity to consent to the sharing of this material may be viewed as a breach of these rights. The UNCRC and ECHR, however, mainly concern themselves with infringement of the state on the rights of citizens. For example, a hospital that used the image of an *incapax* ICU patient without retrospective permission from the patient on its public website would be in breach of Article 8. While it can be argued that it is unwise for families to share images of their relatives in social media, it is unclear what can be done by ICU staff to prevent this happening, other than discussing with families the implications for the patient of the potentially uncontrolled nature of the spread of information and images via social media.

Many devices such as phones, tablets, and laptops allow storage and automatic entry of passwords for websites, including social media websites, and social media apps do not require login details to be entered every time the app is accessed or information is posted. This means that friends and family of patients can post on the social media feeds of the patient to inform their followers of events during the patient's ICU stay. Unless the patient has given explicit permission for this to happen and also administrator rights to those posting, these posts will have been made without permission of the account holder. The Computer Misuse Act (1990)[50] renders it a criminal offence to gain unauthorized access to a computer and cause it to perform any function with intent to secure access to any program or data held in that, or any, computer. Accessing a mobile device or computer in order to modify content on a social media webpage or app could fall under the auspices of this Act. There have been no prosecutions under this Act of a family member of an *incapax* patient who has posted on the social media account of the patient without permission, but the potential illegality of such an act is perhaps another reason why families should be counselled regarding the use of social media in an ICU.

Social media is an increasingly powerful tool for education and communication for healthcare professionals working in intensive care. It is almost inevitable that families of patients lacking capacity will use some form of social media-based communication while their family member is a patient in an ICU, and those of us caring for such patients may need to counsel families on the potential risks of liberal sharing of information in this situation. There are guidelines for registered medical and nursing practitioners using social media, and inappropriate use may result in professional sanctions. Lastly, while social media may provide a tool for education and fast, free sharing of information, it may also be misused as a tool for harassment, and perpetrators of such behavior may face criminal sanction. Social media has increased in popularity and prominence at a rapid rate over the past decade. It is now a permanent feature of the personal lives of the majority of the UK population, and is playing an important part in the professional lives of many healthcare professionals in the intensive care community. Knowledge of the nature of social media, its uses and abuses, should now be considered core knowledge for all those working in our specialty.

References

1. Obar JA, Wildman S. Social media: definition and the governance challenge. Telecommunications Policy 2015 Feb; 39(9):745–750.
2. https://www.statista.com/statistics/264810/number-of-monthly-active-facebook-users-worldwide (accessed 21 December 2019).
3. https://www.statista.com/statistics/282087/number-of-monthly-active-twitter-users (accessed 9 December 2019).
4. Campbell L, Evans Y, Pumper M, Moreno A. Social media use by physicians: a qualitative study of the new frontier of medicine. BMC Medical Informatics and Decision Making. [Internet] 2016 [cited 2 August 2018]; 16(91) doi:10.1186/s12911-016-0327-y (accessed 21 December 2019)
5. OFCOM. *Adult media use and attitudes*. Stationery Office: London, 2017.
6. Bosslet GT, Torke AM, Hickman SE, Terry CL, Helft PR. The patient-doctor relationship and online social networks: results of a national survey. Journal of General Internal Medicine 2011 Oct; 26(10):1168–7426.
7. https://www.bbc.co.uk/news/health-40752061 (accessed 9 December 2019).
8. [2017] EWHC 1909 (Fam) at p11.
9. https://www.theguardian.com/uk-news/2018/apr/28/call-from-god-american-pro-lifers-role-in-alfie-evans-battle?CMP=Share_iOSApp_Other (accessed 9 December 2019).
10. https://www.bbc.co.uk/news/uk-england-merseyside-43746174 (accessed 9 December 2019).
11. https://alderhey.nhs.uk/contact-us/press-office/latest-news/open-letter-chairman-and-chief-executive-alder-hey-childrens-nhs-foundation-trust (accessed 9 December 2019).
12. Munger K. Tweetment effects on the tweeted: experimentally reducing racist harassment. Political Behaviour 2016 Nov; 39(3):629–649.
13. Cheng J, Berstein M, Leskovec J. Anyone can become a troll: causes of trolling behaviour in online discussions. Proceedings of the 2017 ACM conference on computer supported cooperative work and social computing 2017 http://dx.doi.org/10.1145/2998181.2998213 (accessed 4 August 2018).
14. OFCOM. Adult media use and attitudes.
15. http://www.pewinternet.org/2017/07/11/online-harassment-2017/ (accessed 9 December 2019).
16. https://www.bma.org.uk/advice/employment/ethics/social-media-guidance-for-doctors (accessed 9 December 2019).
17. Ibid.

18. https://www.cps.gov.uk/legal-guidance/social-media-guidelines-prosecuting-cases-involving-communications-sent-social-media (accessed 9 December 2019).

19. Suler J. The online disinhibition effect. Cyberpsychology and behaviour 2004 July; 7(3):321–326.

20. Kokolakis S. Privacy attitudes and privacy behaviour; a review of current research on the privacy paradox phenomenon. Computers and Security 2017 Jan; 64(1):122–134.

21. https://www.theguardian.com/uk-news/2016/mar/01/doctor-posted-expletive-filled-twitter-rants-about-patients-tribunal-hears (accessed 9 December 2019).

22. https://www.nursingtimes.net/roles/nurse-managers/nurse-suspended-over-facebook-posts/5062854.article (accessed 9 December 2019).

23. General Medical Council. *Doctors' use of social media*. GMC: London, 2013.

24. General Medical Council. *Good medical practice*. GMC: London, 2013.

25. General Medical Council. *Confidentiality: good practice in handling patient information*. GMC: London, 2017.

26. GMC, *Doctors' use of social media*.

27. Ibid, paragraph 17.

28. http://careers.bmj.com/careers/advice/GMC_defends_guidance_on_social_media_anonymity (accessed 9 December 2019).

29. https://www.facebook.com/notes/general-medical-council-gmc/doctors-use-of-social-media/549553408401395 (accessed 9 December 2019).

30. Nursing and Midwifery Council. *Guidance on using social media responsibly*. NMC: London, 2018.

31. Nursing and Midwifery Council. *The Code: professional standards of practice and behaviour for nurses and midwives (the Code)*. NMC: London, 2015.

32. Nursing and Midwifery Council. *Guidance on using social media responsibly*. NMC: London, 2018.

33. https://www.nhsbt.nhs.uk/get-involved/promoting-donation-hub/download-digital-materials/organ-donation-social-media (accessed 9 December 2019).

34. https://www.sepsis.org/sepsis-awareness-month-toolkit (accessed 21 December 2019).

35. https://hellomynameis.org.uk (accessed 9 December 2019).

36. Shilcutt SK, Silver JK. Social media and advancement of women physicians. New England Journal of Medicine 2018 Jun; 378(24):2342–2345.

37. Campbell et al., Social media use by physicians.

38. https://www.youtube.com/results?search_query=central+line+insertion (accessed 21 December 2019).

39. Khan R, Kashup R, Bhat A, Schulman D, Bruno K, Carrall C. Growth in social media and live-tweeting at major critical care conferences: Twitter analysis of

the past 4 years. Chest [Internet] 2017 [cited 31 July 2018]; 152(suppl4):A547. https://journal.chestnet.org/article/S0012-3692(17)32095-0/fulltext (accessed 21 December 2019).

40. https://www.hon.ch/en/about.html (accessed 21 December 2019).

41. Brulet A, Llorca G, Letrilliart L. Medical wikis dedicated to clinical practice: a systematic review. Journal of Medical Internet Research 2015; 17(2):e48.

42. General Medical Council. *Good medical practice.* GMC: London, 2014.

43. General Medical Council. *Financial and commercial arrangements and conflict of interest.* GMC: London, 2013.

44. https://socialmedia.mayoclinic.org/2017/09/27/online-support-group-informs-uplifts-icu-survivors (accessed 9 December 2019).

45. https://www.facebook.com/groups/icusurvivors (accessed 9 December 2019).

46. https://www.facebook.com/BrightestStarCharity (accessed 9 December 2019).

47. https://www.twitch.tv/p/en-gb/legal/terms-of-service (accessed 9 December 2019).

48. Keith BE, Steinberg S. Parental sharing on the internet. Child privacy in the age of social media and the paediatrician's role. JAMA Pediatrics 2017 May; 171(5): 413–414.

49. https://treaties.un.org/Pages/ViewDetails.aspx?src=IND&mtdsg_no=IV-11&chapter=4&lang=en (accessed 9 December 2019).

50. https://www.legislation.gov.uk/ukpga/1990/18/contents (accessed 9 December 2019).

11

Pandemic Planning after Covid-19

Christopher Danbury, Christopher Newdick, Alex Ruck Keene, and Carl Waldmann

Introduction

What happens when demand for intensive care exceeds the supply of beds available? Rationing intensive care beds happens from time to time,[1] but Covid-19 threatens to create a crisis on a very different scale. This chapter was written as the pandemic was developing in the spring of 2020, when the UK and, indeed, most of the world was in lockdown to minimize social interaction. It grapples with the awful but unavoidable question of rationing intensive care if a situation arrived where not all those who could benefit could be treated. We note, however, that despite the fears for Covid-19, many intensive care departments have not had to ration intensive care beds. The new facilities, named 'NHS Nightingale Hospitals', have not been put to large-scale use and many intensivists are working in much the same way as before. This chapter, therefore, discusses the planning necessary to respond to a pandemic—which has yet to become necessary in the NHS. We discuss the law and ethics surrounding this emergency in its immediate aftermath, knowing that further research and learning will continue to emerge. Given the constraints of time, we cannot reflect on the impact of Covid-19, the responses to it, or the reforms that become necessary as a result. Our intention is necessarily less ambitious. It is simply to highlight the major questions raised by the crisis and some plausible solutions.

Our discussion is divided into three sections: (1) the nature and extent of the demand for intensive care and the government's response (up until April 2020), (2) the necessity for a procedural framework for decision making to promote transparency, fairness and consistency, and (3) the models of clinical triage to achieve the best results.

Nature and extent of demand for intensive care

Prior to the Covid-19 outbreak, the UK had a limited critical care capacity. Rhodes et al.[2] showed that the number of critical care beds was 6.6 per 100,000 population. This compared with 11.6 in France and 29.2 in Germany. Within Europe, this placed the UK in 24th position out of the 31 countries studied. The number of acute beds fell over the preceding years. As the King's Fund has said: 'The total number of NHS hospital beds in England ... has more than halved over the past 30 years, from around 299,000 in 1987/88 to 141,000 in 2018/9, while the number of patients treated has increased significantly.'[3] Critical care provision increased in the past decade, rising from 3,679 adult critical care beds in March 2011[4] to 4,122 in February 2020[5], a rise of 14%. At the same time, the population in the UK is expected to increase by 5.9% between mid-2016 and mid-2026, an average annual increase of ~1% as the number of older people is expected to double. Both will have an impact on demand for critical care services. The net effect of decreasing numbers of acute beds and increasing population puts a disproportionate stress on critical care services within the acute general hospital where there is a projected annual 4% increase in demand for intensive care. Measured over the longer period, this 4% annual increase in demand would have merited a 42% increase in critical care provision over the past decade; and this demonstrates the stress that critical care services in the UK were exposed to going into the Covid-19 pandemic. Patient flow through acute hospitals has been compounded by limitations in community care and the fact that hospital beds are unavailable by reason of patients who cannot be discharged home, or to other institutions, and are therefore 'blocking' the timely discharge of an ICU patient back to ward care. Even allowing for these statistics, the extra critical care capacity would not be sufficient to respond to a major pandemic where it would be necessary to allow for an increase of three or four times capacity to meet the surge or peak in demand.

Most hospitals plan for a pandemic by cancelling non-urgent surgical work and using theatre space for intensive care patients. This has enabled a temporary increase in critical care provision by three or four times the base provision. With respect to ventilators, on 13 April, it was reported that the NHS had access to 10,120 ventilators, an increase from 8,175 in mid-March 2020. More were received from countries such as Germany and China, and on 5 April Health Secretary Matt Hancock set a target of 18,000 ventilators[6] and the government also urged manufacturers to divert their energies into producing ventilators to a common standard.[7] But the scheme was not a success: the Faculty of Intensive Care Medicine said the standard was insufficient to meet the complex needs of Covid-19 patients[8] and there were regulatory and logistical difficulties. There was also concern about the risks of using untrained staff[9] and, in the end, demand for ventilator support was less than anticipated.

Unsurprisingly, perhaps, at such short notice, as knowledge of Covid-19 was developing, the scheme was overwhelmed by unintended complications.

There is a minimal private critical care provision in the UK. It is concentrated in London, where 102 beds have been identified,[10] and was quickly discounted as a potential resource by NHS providers because it would dilute the necessary manpower. Intensive care has had to adapt by using different staff to patient ratios and by forming teams for specific care such as intubation, tracheostomy, line insertion, and proning; the latter procedure aids the invasive ventilation of the very challenging respiratory physiology produced by the SARS-CoV-2.

At the time of writing, the resources in the private sector have yet to be utilized effectively. However, it is anticipated that elective surgery will be decanted to this area to minimize the inevitable increase in waiting lists that Covid-19 will bring. The temporary Nightingale hospitals have not, at the time of writing, received significant numbers of patients. For instance, the original venue at the ExCel Centre ostensibly has space for 4,000 ventilated patients. We assume a dilution of staff to patient ratios by four times usual practice to one nurse to four patients, one junior doctor to 24 patients, and one consultant to 48 patients. To supply a functioning 24/7 rota, seven healthcare professionals need to be available at each of these tiers. On this basis, to staff the ExCel NHS Nightingale would require 7,000 nurses, 1,167 junior doctors, and 584 consultant intensive care physicians—at a time when there are 641 whole time equivalent intensive care consultants and fewer than 2,000 intensive care doctors in the country.[11] Clearly, these long-standing capacity constraints may have adverse impact elsewhere, and we hope that these facilities will not be needed and that the existing critical care network can continue to treat critically ill patients with all diseases, including Covid-19.

Procedural framework for decision making

Why is a procedural framework necessary?

Reasonable doctors will respond differently to the rationing crisis provoked by Covid-19. Some might insist on their strict Hippocratic commitment to individual patients; in this case, each would receive the best care possible even though such an approach would not save the largest number of patients. Others might adopt a communitarian approach by compromising individual care to promote the greatest health of the greatest number, so as to achieve a broader social objective. Another might give priority to essential workers like clinicians and those in care homes. By contrast, Italian guidelines suggested a simple age cut-off for admission to ICU.[12] Yet others may insist that individual doctors should never make triage decisions because 'they are grounded in public health ethics, not clinical ethics' and, instead, 'a triage team … should make allocation decisions.'[13] Clearly, without a consistent framework, clinical decisions would be inconsistent and might appear unfair. Note that, at the macro-level, when clinical commissioning groups allocate resources, the NHS is required to be open and transparent about its procedures and, we believe, the same principle should apply here, in intensive care.

The procedural framework promotes transparency, fairness, and consistency—namely, that every decision should be made against a background of agreed and stable values. Rationing is lawful, *provided* it is undertaken reasonably and fairly. Judicial review has never guaranteed individual patients substantive rights of access to care, regardless of its cost and impact on other patients. Instead, rationing is lawful provided it is undertaken rationally, in a way that gives proportionate weight to the relevant circumstances, including the needs of others. As the Court of Appeal said in the case of a girl whose father sought a 'last chance' treatment for leukaemia that was expensive and unlikely to be effective or to serve the girl's best interests:

> … in a perfect world any treatment which a patient, or a patient's family, sought would be provided if doctors were willing to give it, no matter how much it cost, particularly when a life was potentially at stake. It would however be shutting one's eyes to the real world if the court were to proceed on the basis that we do live in such a world.… Difficult and agonizing judgments have to be made as to how a limited budget is best allocated to the maximum advantage of the maximum number of patients. That is not a judgment the court can make.[14]

The same approach applies to resource challenges arising from Covid-19, as was recognized in a decision in early April 2020,[15] in which the court granted an injunction requiring a patient with mental health difficulties to leave a bed in an acute hospital because that bed was urgently required for Covid-19 patients. The court said:

> In some circumstances, a hospital may have to decide which of two patients, A or B, has a better claim to a bed, or a better claim to a bed in a particular unit, even ceasing to provide in-patient care to one of them to leave will certainly cause extreme distress or will give rise to significant risks to that patient's health or even life.[16]

Within this proviso, the ethical framework should state how fairness and consistency between patients should be achieved. To leave this weighty decision to doctors alone would expose patients to the risk of differing responses depending on who was treating them. Separating triage coordination from the delivery of care to individual patients also reduces the potential for moral distress among treating clinicians.[17] We recommend, therefore, maintaining a clear distinction between the role of individual clinicians dealing with the patients before them, and the corporate responsibility of the Trust for allocating resources.

Who should develop the procedural framework?

There is an argument that government itself should recommend such a procedural framework—for example, a 'Covid-19 ethical framework for decision making.' As we write, judicial review proceedings are being considered to urge the government to do exactly this. Government, however, has always resisted this invitation. Cynics will say it associates government too closely with the adverse impact of successive governments' failure to fund the NHS to levels comparable to our European partners. Equally, government may respond that these functions have always been delegated to local health authorities and hospitals because they are better placed to allocate their resources to local needs than a remote government in London.

As we write, therefore, the responsibility for triage coordination—or at least triage *preparation*—has fallen to hospitals, but, because hospitals have to coordinate with each other to maximize bed capacity, they should also cooperate with one another, including by agreeing a common framework of procedures, if possible, and some form of oversight of hospital activity at regional level.[18]

Which procedures are involved?

There are a number of procedural considerations and we discuss: (a) triage coordinators, (b) triage oversight, (c) conversations with patients and relatives, and (d) disagreement between doctors and patients or their relatives.

(a) Triage coordinators

The objective of rationing intensive care within a system of procedures is to encourage decision making that serves the interests of the community as a whole and responds to patients' needs fairly, equally, and consistently. Hospital triage coordinators provide a consistent reference point for decision making. There should be clear line management from the hospital triage-coordinator to the hospital board. Although the individual does not necessarily have to be medically qualified, the clinical director for critical care would be a logical choice for this individual. Triage coordinators should guide and advise colleagues—for example, as to which patients should be moved from one level of care to another; which patients should not be offered care in the interests of admitting others; or who should be removed from intensive care to receive palliative care. The job of distinguishing different categories of patient is likely to be emotionally demanding. For these reasons, hospitals should appoint a team of coordinators to share the burden. While this carries the cost of withdrawing experienced clinicians from their patients, the long-term advantage is obvious. So long as coherent clinical criteria have been developed within this framework, fair, equal, and consistent decision making will be encouraged. Given the incomplete and uncertain clinical evidence surrounding many patients, decision making is less likely to be undertaken by individual doctors at risk of complaint for deviating from the practice adopted by their colleagues.

Triage at the regional level will also be desirable to coordinate activity when individual hospitals run short of beds and seek capacity elsewhere. As the National Institute for Health and Care Excellence (NICE) suggested in its COVID-19 rapid guideline:

> Hospitals should discuss the sharing of resources and the transfer of patients between units, including units in other hospitals, to ensure the best use of critical care within the NHS. . . . Data on the availability of critical care beds should be made available to critical care decision makers and operational management team to facilitate the sharing of resources.[19]

To the extent that doctors in an entire region can mobilize together in this way, resources are likely to be put to optimum and consistent use. Even more extreme, but potentially more valuable, were the steps taken to create very large field hospitals to serve as the ICU hub for a particular region, the first being the ExCel NHS Nightingale for London, created out of the ExCel conference centre. We have expressed concern, above, about diverting a finite body of clinical expertise from other hospitals, but coordination at regional level is likely to be put resources to optimum and consistent use. Regular exchange of information between the local and regional levels will be important. Regional triage may also be a good location for disseminating knowledge and learning to improve care. But doubtless this too absorbs colleagues' time and skill and must be balanced against the benefit to be gained from devoting themselves to patient care.

(b) Triage oversight

Triage coordination is not just the responsibility of individual doctors, or co-ordinating teams. It is principally the responsibility of the Trust itself, for two reasons. First, it fulfils the Trust's responsibility to allocate scarce resources according to transparent criteria for determining access to intensive care and treatments within critical care, and (if needs be) discontinuation of care. Intensivists should feed into and update the criteria, but should not have ul-timate responsibility for their content. It will, at the same time, ensure that the resource allocation decisions are made with the support of healthcare profes-sionals with expert knowledge and skills in critical care.

The second objective of 'triage oversight' is to encourage procedural justice. A helpful formulation of this function can be found in this (US) description (not all of which can be directly applied to the present context):

> In order to ensure "procedural justice," a standardized and equitable practice that conforms to the rules in place, any triage operation should be regularly and repeatedly evaluated to guarantee that the process has been followed fairly. This evaluation process will promote medical provider compliance; eliminate admin-istrator, governmental, or physician overrule (special pleadings or "favors"); and facilitate consistency. Owing to the critical illness of patients and the limitations of the scarce resource(s), this evaluation process will need to be efficient and frequent. Direct appeals to the triage procedure may be impractical based on the urgency with which the allocation decision must be made. Individual phys-icians, administrators, or government officials should not be able to overrule a "good faith" decision made by a triage officer in compliance with the triage pro-cess. Because all patients will share the same pool of resources, the standard of care and triage process should apply to all patients, whether their condition is directly attributable to the mass casualty event or results from other underlying pathology or circumstances. If there is a challenge to procedural justice (ie, the process was not followed according to established criteria), then an appeal is indicated.[20]

Procedural justice is a critical aspect of the legal obligations imposed upon the Trust as a public body. Neither the National Health Service Act 2006, the Human Rights Act 1998 nor the Equality Act 2010 (nor indeed any other le-gislation, nor case-law[21]) require Trusts to provide access to critical care, or specific treatments within critical care, if they are not, in fact, available. This is so whether the patient has capacity to participate in the decisions being made or not.[22] However, what is required is that the Trust has in place procedures to enable decisions to be made in a way that is rational, accountable, transparent and non-discriminatory.

For example, a triage oversight board might discharge its functions by way of regular meetings to consider a sample of decisions taken in the previous days, receiving data in terms of how the processes and criteria are working in practice, and whether either require change. We note the final sentence of the extract above, which recommends the creation of an appeal procedure. Perhaps a regional oversight board could also serve as an internal appeals structure, but time will often preclude such a process and to promise a procedure that is no more than a sham invites severe criticism. Nonetheless, within the oversight of the board, there is merit in having a pool of experienced clinicians (including those with expertise in complex decision making), from whom triage teams could seek assistance with the resolution of disagreement and uncertainty.

(c) Candour with patients and relatives

Doctors should normally discuss end of life care candidly with their patients. In *R (Tracey) v Cambridge University Hospital NHS Foundation Trust*, the Court of Appeal balanced the need for candour with the distress it may cause to patients. Risk of distress increases when patients who were previously fit and strong are overwhelmed unexpectedly by illness. In *Tracey*, the hospital argued that non-disclosure could be justified to save the patient the distress of a discussion about withholding life-support treatment. However, the court rejected the argument. Lord Dyson said that the balance continues to favour disclosure given the importance of the decision:

> Prima facie, the patient is entitled to know that such an important clinical decision has been taken. The fact that the clinician considers that CPR will not work means that the patient cannot require him to provide it. It does not, however, mean that the patient is not entitled to know that the clinical decision has been taken.

However, Lord Dyson also recognized that:

> Many patients may find it distressing to discuss the question whether CPR should be withheld from them in the event of a cardio-respiratory arrest. If however the clinician forms the view that the patient will not suffer harm if she is consulted, the fact that she may find the topic distressing is unlikely to make it inappropriate to involve her. I recognise that these are difficult issues which require clinicians to make

sensitive decisions sometimes in very stressful circumstances. I would add that the court should be very slow to find that such decisions, if conscientiously taken, violate a patient's rights under article 8 of the Convention.[23]

Although we recognize the time constraints imposed on clinical staff, we do not believe there is a compelling reason to depart from this principle of candour in the circumstances of Covid-19. None of the guidance suggests the contrary.[24] Needless to say, none of this should compromise the care and compassion every patient should receive, whatever the decision about the nature of the care available.

Should relatives also be involved in this discussion? Patients are entitled to keep the decision-making process confidential if they wish, but, absent an express statement of this nature and bearing in mind that intensive care patients may have limited capacity to discuss their treatment, doctors might reasonably assume that patients are content for relatives to be involved.[25] Consultation, however, also creates the possibility of disagreement; indeed, there is normally a right to seek a second opinion. As the Court of Appeal said in *Tracey*, 'if the patient is not told that the clinician has made a DNACPR decision, he will be deprived of the opportunity of seeking a second opinion.'[26] As discussed in Chapter 6, the Supreme Court in *An NHS Trust v Y* decided that the involvement of the court to test the lawfulness of a decision to withdraw active treatment is not required when there is agreement between patient (or their relatives) and clinicians:

> where all the proper procedures have been observed and there is no doubt about what is in the best interests of the patient, there is much to be said for enabling the family and the patient to spend their last days together without the burden and distraction, and possibly expense, of court proceedings.[27]

Equally, the right to a second opinion clearly recognizes the possibility of a disagreement about the best course of action.

(d) Disagreement between doctors and patients or relatives

In *Y*, the Supreme Court was clear that differences of opinion between clinicians or relatives should normally be resolved by a court:

> If, at the end of the medical process, it is apparent that the way forward is finely balanced, or there is a difference of medical opinion, or a lack of agreement to a proposed course of action from those with an interest in the patient's welfare, a court application can and should be made.[28]

Covid-19 imposes considerable strain on this principle. Given the numbers of patients receiving intensive care, and the unexpected and sudden nature of their admission, one might expect larger numbers than usual to request a second opinion, some of which may end in disagreement (although, to date, it seems that serious disagreements have been remarkably few). In the way of things, time will not permit counsel or judges to argue and adjudicate about these cases and the expectations in *Y* of legal proceedings will often be impossible to achieve. 'Second opinion' procedures should be routine in any event to reassure patients and relatives so far as possible about end of life decisions.[29] Acknowledging the constraints on the time available during the crisis, a procedural framework of expectations should encourage senior doctors always to be available at short notice to offer a second opinion about Covid-19 patients. Triage coordinators will contribute to this role and help to resolve many of the differences of opinion.

> But what happens to the remaining cases when these 'second opinion' procedures cannot bring the parties to agreement? NICE advises clinicians simply to: [s]top critical care treatment when it is no longer considered able to achieve the desired overall goals (outcomes). Record the decision and the discussion with family and carers, the patient (if possible) or an independent mental capacity advocate (if appropriate).[30]

This does not confront the problem of disagreement discussed in *Y*. One solution may be available from the Supreme Court in *Aintree University Hospital NHS Foundation Trust v James*,[31] concerning patients who wish treatment in intensive care to continue, despite the contrary judgment of their doctors. In *James*, the Supreme Court laid down a *subjective* approach to assessing the patient's best interests that respects the patient's wish for treatment to continue. Recall that Mr James had been an intensive care patient for many months before he died. Clearly, however, in the strained circumstances of the pandemic crisis, an uncritical approach to patients' subjective wishes that disregarded their condition could have a significant adverse impact on other patients deprived of intensive care as a consequence, for whom intensive care could otherwise save their lives. How should this tension be resolved? In *James,* the Supreme Court acknowledged two circumstances when we, as patients, 'cannot always have what we want':[32] this is when: (a) no doctor is prepared to continue active treatment because none consider it to be in our best interests, and (b) those responsible for allocating finite resources are applying a rational and legitimate policy that excludes patients who fall within the category concerned. The Supreme Court in *N v ACCG*[33] subsequently reinforced the message that the Court of Protection: 'only has power to take a decision that P himself could have taken? It has no greater power to oblige others to do what is best than P would have himself. This must mean that, just like P, the court can only choose between the "available options." '[34]

Provided the policy is lawful applying conventional judicial review principles, neither the Court of Protection nor the Administrative Court has authority to contradict the legitimate discretion of the public authority.[35] This reasoning, particularly in (b), may help resolve cases in which agreement between intensive care clinicians and patients or their relatives is impossible. Such a result, without the usual judicial scrutiny, is troubling, and depends on the foundation of fair, reasonable and consistent triage procedures. Nevertheless, a proper procedural framework should be sufficient to rebalance the debate toward maximizing survival of as many patients as possible from a pandemic as a legitimate objective.

Clinical triage to achieve the best results

Within this procedural framework, what guidance should doctors receive to distinguish between patients? Pandemics challenge traditional Hippocratic notions of reasonable care. When patient demand exceeds the beds or ventilators available, unfamiliar choices are required. 'A public health emergency creates a need to transition from individual patient-focused clinical care to a population-oriented public health approach . . . '[36] As the British Medical Association says, 'health professionals may be obliged to withdraw treatment from some patients to enable treatment of other patients with a higher survival probability.'[37] As we discussed earlier, in this changed environment, clinical 'instinct' will vary, but inconsistent approaches appear unfair and unreasonable. Within the ethical, procedural framework, on what common clinical criteria should decision making take place? Bear in mind that resource pressures will differ from place to place. Patients may present with multiple illnesses, particularly those who have long-term conditions (for instance, end-stage renal failure), and individual circumstances are hugely variable so that diagnosis and prognosis are often uncertain. And pandemic pressures on beds limit the time available for reflection. Given these variables, how can we devise constructive criteria to guide clinicians' decisions?

Unacceptable discrimination

Start with the obvious: discrimination on irrelevant grounds such as race, sex, gender, religion, nationality, or age is always unacceptable. Space precludes extensive discussion of the Equality Act 2010. However, let us pause on the question of age, which is a 'protected characteristic' under the Act. How should clinicians respond to guidelines that refer to age as a relevant criterion for rationing? Age may be a permissible consideration provided that the decision maker can demonstrate that it is 'a proportionate means of achieving a legitimate aim'. Put another way, provided the decision maker can show why age is a relevant factor in the decision, then it will not amount to discrimination. For example, the Belgian Society of Intensive Care recommends that elderly residents in retirement homes should not normally be admitted to intensive care because it would be 'disproportionate'.[38] But this may be too blunt a measure because many dependent residents look after themselves and require low levels of support. Indeed, such a response in the UK might contravene the 2010 Act for seeking a legitimate aim by *dis*proportionate means.

Blanket 'exclusionary' criteria may also be criticized because they exclude patients' individual circumstances. For example, age by itself is never likely to be appropriate. A more 'inclusive' approach is reflected by the Clinical Frailty Scale (CFS), recommended by NICE.[39] The CFS has a nine-point scale to assess a range of considerations and whether patients will benefit from intensive care (with those most vulnerable scoring highest on the scale). But even this may be too blunt a tool. When, in March 2020, NICE recommended use of the CFS, it was criticized by MENCAP for being too generic.[40] Scale 7 of the CFS describes patients who are: 'Severely Frail—Completely Dependent for Personal Care [but] ... not at high risk of dying ... ' Shortly afterwards, and following the threat of judicial review proceedings, NICE acknowledged it had failed to indicate that not all patients on the same point of the scale should be treated the same. For example, patients with stable mental illness should not be treated in the same way as dependent adults whose conditions are progressively deteriorating. For example, treatment decisions should not disfavour those who are disabled simply by reason of their disability. Thus, the NICE guideline was amended to read:

> Be aware of the limitations of using the CFS as the sole assessment of frailty. The CFS should not be used in younger people, people with stable long-term disabilities (for example, cerebral palsy), learning disabilities or autism. An individualised assessment is recommended in all cases where the CFS is not appropriate.

The CFS must be understood, therefore, as a general guide to be applied to each patient's individual circumstances.

Are patient scoring systems helpful?

A more condition-specific tool is explored by the University of Pittsburgh Department of Critical Care Medicine in the Sequential Organ Failure Assessment (SOFA) scoring system. The Pittsburgh guideline candidly states that '[c]onsistent with accepted standards during public health emergencies, a goal of the allocation framework is to achieve the most good for populations of patients.'[41] Patients are assessed on a scale of 1 to 8 (with a higher score representing patients most at risk), and 'patients who are more likely to survive with intensive care are prioritized over patients who are less likely to survive with intensive care.' Points are awarded according to the severity of disease and the likelihood of death. Examples of conditions with a moderate score are 'major comorbidities associated with decreased long-term survival'—for example, moderate Alzheimer's disease, malignancy with less than 10 years' survival, heart failure (NY Heart Association Class III), moderately severe chronic lung disease, and end-stage renal disease in patients under 75. By contrast, conditions attracting a higher score are 'life limiting comorbidities commonly associated with survival of less than one year', including severe Alzheimer's disease, cancer being treated with only palliative care, Class IV heart failure, severe chronic lung disease with evidence of frailty, and end-stage renal disease in patients older than 75.

Returning to the example of the Belgian Society of Intensive Care, a Sequential Organ Failure Assessment (SOFA) score may be a better way of weighing the clinical merits of residents in a care home and produce a more defensible conclusion. The Pittsburgh guidance continues that patients should be reassessed regularly: 'if there are patients in the queue ... patients who upon reassessment show *substantial deterioration* as evidenced by worsening SOFA scores or overall clinical judgment should have critical care withdrawn.'[42] More difficult is when beneficial treatment for one slowly recovering patient deprives others from treatment 'that could lead to better outcomes for a larger number ... '[43] Should treatment be withdrawn here too? These are most troubling decisions for doctors. Clearly, as we discussed earlier, there is a duty of candour and relatives should be involved in the process of withdrawal, but not to the extent that they may override the clinical decision (as is clear from the case of *MB*, above).

Trusting clinical judgment

Any scoring system has limitations. SOFA or the modified APACHE II score used by ICNARC[44] depend on a retrospective analysis of the physiological and laboratory data. This is not very useful in 'real time' clinical practice. The National Early Warning Score (NEWS)[45] and NEWS2 are useful, but not disease specific, and early reports suggest limitations with use in Covid-19. By contrast, some hospitals are using a simpler, three-criteria model based on high, medium, and low priority. Patients with highest priority are those most likely to make a rapid recovery. Low priority is given to patients with the lowest probability of doing so. Priority is given to patients according to their capacity to recover and the speed with which they are likely to do so. These judgments are informed by evidence of patients' comorbidities (as with SOFA), but patients are not assigned a 'score'. Instead, doctors are responsible for applying flexible criteria within their own judgment, together with their triage teams and coordinators, in the light of each patient's individual circumstances and the resources available. The advantage of such a system is that it recognizes that scoring systems are not entirely 'objective' because each score is an exercise of clinical judgment, often based on incomplete evidence. Although experienced clinicians show a close correlation with the predictions of objective scoring systems such as APACHE II or SOFA,[46] doctors' predictions of outcome often correlate poorly with *actual* outcomes: doctors have unconscious biases of their own, like everyone else, which may affect objective decision making. Arguably, this three-criteria approach is an acceptably candid mechanism for responding to the pressures on resources. Proper records of every such decision must be maintained so that we can understand how and why each decision was made. And, of course, patients not admitted to intensive care will always receive proper, compassionate, palliative care.

Opinions will differ whether a three-criteria model of this nature can adequately accommodate the many clinical variations between patients. Some will say it promotes flexibility at the expense of consistency and, therefore, lacks transparency. Each point on the spectrum of alternatives presents risks and benefits, and no system is perfect. The system must be workable at a day-to-day level and be sufficiently transparent to provide a reasonably fair and consistent framework for decision making. Given the time constraints, provided some such system is in place, perhaps allowance can be made one way or the other when judgments differ.

Sometimes decisions will be required when distinguishing between one patient's score and another is impossible. In circumstances where fine distinctions between patients are impossible, the Belgian guidelines suggest the 'first come first served' principle. The Pittsburgh guidance would give extra weight to essential clinical staff and younger patients. Others give credit to 'first responders'.[47] In other cases, SOFA may fail to distinguish patients whom clinicians may have proper reason to consider are, in fact, different. Take the example of two patients with the same score, one of whom has a chronic condition, the other is suffering acute change. Despite their identical scores, many clinicians would prioritize the latter. Scoring systems, therefore, cannot remove reasonable disagreement and it is mistaken to believe they can generate a 'correct' or 'objective' solution. Indeed, it may be that, for all the energy invested in developing fair and constructive scoring systems, the disputes that may arise later will continue to be resolved on the basis of reasonable, well-informed and consistent care, and good faith. In this case, the *Bolam* principle will continue to play a significant role, albeit in its 'hard-look' form in which the courts are willing to probe and scrutinize the rationale for decision making.[48]

Let us not forget also the goal of public health to reduce the spread of disease. Scoring systems do not work well for populations of people. Public health must focus on preventive care and the groups of citizens most at risk. 'Protecting health may mean prioritizing resources for people in confined settings (such as homeless shelters, prisons and nursing homes), where the virus can spread rapidly ... [and] to areas experiencing localized outbreaks.'[49] Attention rightly focuses on essential workers, such as carers in care homes, those operating public transport, and delivery drivers. But in the allocation of personal protective equipment, how would a scoring system compare their needs with those working in hospitals?

Conclusion

As we conclude this chapter, there is hope that the worst of the pandemic in the NHS is passing, although it continues to develop elsewhere globally. Local intensive care units (ICUs) have largely managed the additional demands on their beds and the Nightingale hospitals have not been confronted with heavy demand. Perhaps, therefore, the most difficult and unfamiliar scenario of rationing threatened by Covid-19 will not happen, although there is a residual fear of a second wave of resurgence of the virus and we do not know what the final mortality will be. We draw attention, however, to two aspects of the experience of responses to Covid-19 that raise concern.

First, whether out of a mistaken aim to ensure that supply was only matched by 'true' demand, a misunderstanding of the law,[50] or otherwise, it appeared that significant numbers of individuals were having decisions made as to resuscitation without any form of consultation; in other cases, it appeared that individuals were being pressured into signing their own DNACPR notices.[51] Many such individuals were elderly, but did not have specific disabilities. In other cases, it appeared that judgments were being made that (for example) CPR should not be attempted because patients had, for instance, a learning disability. National bodies sought to take remedial action,[52] but, at the time of writing, it remained unclear whether this would have a material effect.

Second, the concentration on the potential for triage meant that there was—perhaps—inadequate recognition that it was in the interests of clinicians, and the public, to have in place clear support mechanisms to enable the making and recording of complex decisions in the face of stretched, but not overwhelmed, resource, what we have called a 'procedural framework'. Absent such support mechanisms, there was—and remains—a risk of triage by stealth: in other words, decisions being made by clinicians unduly motivated by concerns as to resource. More generally, support mechanisms will also be required to enable clinicians to navigate a new world in which it is necessary, first, to balance their duties to patients with risks to themselves from inadequate resources in the form of personal protective equipment,[53] and, second, to recognize the impact of prioritizing critical care on the options for patients in other treatment settings for whom resources have diminished.

We have considered the ways in which healthcare systems could respond to the pandemic, both by way of procedural structures and triage criteria. Looking to the future, inquiries will naturally examine the causes of the crisis, both remote and local, how well we responded, and the reforms required. Perhaps it will force us to reconsider the costs to the NHS of welfare austerity since 2010, which has so reduced the numbers of hospital beds, doctors, nurses, and community care staff. The crisis highlights the need to reflect on the resource requirements of a comprehensive NHS, especially when compared with the capacity of similar services in other developed nations. It also reminds us, if we needed reminding, of the threat of a global pandemic, which we understand, but have done so little to counter. Should nations cooperate more openly with one another to minimize the dangers, what is the role of the World Health Organization and to what extent should the phenomenon of globalization be modified to reduce the risk? There are many questions, but, in the light of this experience, many will wish to contribute to the debate that follows the long shadow of Covid-19.

Notes

1. Metcalfe et al. speculate that 2,100–2,500 preventable deaths annually may have been caused in the 1990s by lack of access to intensive care beds. See Metcalfe MA, Sloggett A, McPherson K. (1997). Mortality among appropriately referred patients refused admission to intensive-care units. *Lancet*, **350**, 7.

2. Rhodes AP, Ferdinande H, Flaatten B, et al. (2012, 10 July). The variability of critical care bed numbers in Europe. *Intensive Care Medicine*, **38(10)**, 1647–53. https://doi.org/10.1007/s00134-012-2627-8 (accessed 11 June 2020).

3. The King's Fund (2020, 26 March). NHS hospital bed numbers. https://www.kingsfund.org.uk/publications/nhs-hospital-bed-numbers (accessed 11 June 2020).

4. https://www.england.nhs.uk/statistics/wp-content/uploads/sites/2/2013/04/MSitRep_March_2010-11.xls (accessed 11 June 2020).

5. https://www.england.nhs.uk/statistics/wp-content/uploads/sites/2/2020/04/MSitRep-Timeseries-February-2020-alHTC.xls (accessed 11 June 2020).

6. See *Coronavirus: Ventilator availability in the UK*, House of Commons Briefing Paper 8902, 27 April 2020, from which this paragraph is taken. See UK's new ventilators still awaiting regulatory green light, *Financial Times* (13 April 2020); China sends 300 ventilators to UK as hospital runs out of oxygen fighting coronavirus, *Daily Telegraph* (4 April 2020); Matt Hancock, Outdoor exercise could be banned if people flout rules, *The Andrew Marr Show*, BBC (5 April 2020).

7. See Department for Business, Energy & Industrial Strategy (2020, 16 March). Call for businesses to help make NHS ventilators, and Department of Health & Social Care (2020, 20 March). Rapidly manufactured ventilator system specification. Dyson is reported to have invested £20 million in ventilator production that was not required, see the speech: Johnson's triumphalist moments risk angering NHS workers, *The Guardian* (28 April 2020).

8. See comment of Dr Alison Pittard, Dean of the Faculty of Intensive Care Medicine, Ventilator standards set out for UK makers 'of no use' to Covid patients, *Financial Times* (15 April 2020).

9. Covid-19 ventilator appeal 'pointless' without staff and other kit, *Nursing Times* (16 March 2020).

10. https://www.laingbuisson.com/shop/private-acute-healthcare-central-london-market-report-6-ed/ (accessed 11 June 2020).

11. https://digital.nhs.uk/data-and-information/publications/statistical/nhs-workforce-statistics (accessed 11 June 2020).

12. Italian Society of Anesthesia, Analgesia, Resuscitation and Intensive Care (SIAARTI) (2020, 16 March). *Clinical ethics recommendations for the allocation of intensive care treatments in exceptional, resource-limited circumstances—Version 1*. The age cut-off was proposed in paragraph 3.

13. Belgian Society of Intensive Care Medicine (2020, 18 March). *Ethical principles concerning proportionality of critical care during the COVID-19 pandemic: advice by the Belgian Society of Intensive Care Medicine*, 3.

14. *R v Cambridge DHA, ex p B* [1995] 2 All ER 129, 137.

15. *University College London Hospitals NHS Foundation Trust v MB* [2020] 882 (QB). Arrangements were in place so that the patient would receive the NHS care that she required for her mental health condition outside hospital.

16. Paragraph 55.
17. See, for example, White DB, Lo B. (2020). A framework for rationing ventilators and critical care beds during the COVID-19 pandemic. *JAMA*. Published online 27 March https://doi:10.1001/jama.2020.5046 (accessed 11 June 2020).
18. See Christian M, Sprung C, King M, et al. (2014). Triage: care of the critically ill and injured during pandemics and disasters: CHEST consensus statement. *Chest*, **146**, e615.
19. National Institute for Health and Care Excellence (NICE) (2020). *COVID-19 rapid guideline: critical care in adults*, NG159, paras 5.3–5.4. .
20. Conclusions of a Task Force for Mass Critical Care Summit meeting convened in Chicago in 2007: https://www.sciencedirect.com/science/article/pii/S0012369215327811 (accessed 11 June 2020).
21. See in particular, *R (B) v Cambridge Health Authority* [1995] EWCA Civ 43.
22. See *N v ACCG* [2017] UKSC 22.
23. *R (Tracey) v Cambridge University Hospital NHS Foundation Trust* [2014] EWCA Civ 822, [54]–[55].
24. See, for example, https://beta.bma.org.uk/advice-and-support/covid-19/ethics/covid-19-ethical-issue (accessed 11 June 2020).
25. Of course, the restrictions on access to wards curtail normal conversations and these may have to be conducted remotely.
26. *R (Tracey) v Cambridge University Hospital NHS Foundation Trust* [2014] EWCA Civ 822, [55].
27. *An NHS Trust v Y* [2018] UKSC 46 [121].
28. Ibid., [126], per Lady Black.
29. *Decisions Relating to Cardiopulmonary Resuscitation* (2016), 3rd edition, 1st revision). Guidance from the British Medical Association, the Resuscitation Council and the Royal College of Nursing: http://resus.org.uk/dnacpr/decisions-relating-to-cpr (accessed 11 June 2020).
30. National Institute for Health and Care Excellence (NICE) (2020). *COVID-19 rapid guideline: critical care in adults*, NG159, para 3.3. .
31. *Aintree University Hospital NHS Foundation Trust v James* [2013]. UKSC 67.
32. Ibid., [45], per Lady Hale.
33. [2017] UKSC 22.
34. *MN* at [35]. See also *PW v Chelsea And Westminster Hospital NHS Foundation Trust & Ors* [2018] EWCA Civ 1067 at [97].
35. For a fuller discussion, see Newdick and Danbury in this volume on 'Promoting the Best Possible Death'.
36. US Centers for Disease Control and Prevention (2011). *Ethical considerations for decision making regarding allocation of mechanical ventilation during a severe influenza pandemic or other public health emergency*, 7.
37. British Medical Association (2020). *COVID-19—Ethical issues. A guidance note*.
38. Belgian Society of Intensive Care Medicine (March 2020). *Ethical principles concerning proportionality of critical care during the COVID-19 pandemic: advice by the Belgian Society of IC medicine*.
39. National Institute for Health and Care Excellence (NICE) (2020). *COVID-19 rapid guideline: critical care in adults*, NG159, paras 5.3–5.4. .
40. See 'Mencap respond to NICE COVID-19 guidance' (2 April 2020). https://www.mencap.org.uk/press-release/mencap-responds-deeply-troubling-new-nice-covid-19-guidance (accessed 11 June 2020).

41. University of Pittsburgh (2020). *Allocation of scarce critical care resources during a public health emergency*, 5. See also, Lee Daugherty Biddison E, Faden R, Gwon H, et al. (2018). Too many patients ... a framework to guide statewide allocation of scarce mechanical ventilation during disasters. *Chest*. https://ccm.pitt.edu/sites/default/files/UnivPittsburgh_ModelHospitalResourcePolicy_2020_04_15.pdf (accessed 18 June 2020).

42. No legal or ethical distinction exists between withholding and withdrawing inappropriate care. See *Airedale NHS Trust v Bland* [1993] 1 All ER 821 and Wilkinson D, Savulescu J. (2014). A costly separation between withdrawing and withholding treatment in intensive care. *Bioethics* **28**, 127, discussing the cost of inconsistent clinical practice.

43. British Medical Association (2020). *COVID-19—Ethical Issues. A Guidance Note*. British Medical Association.

44. Harrison David A, Parry Gareth J, Carpenter James R, et al. (2007). A new risk prediction model for critical care: the Intensive Care National Audit & Research Centre (ICNARC) model. *Critical Care Medicine* **35(4)**, June, 1091–8. https://doi.org/10.1097/01.CCM.0000259468.24532.44 (accessed 11 June 2020).

45. Royal College of Physicians of London (2012). *National Early Warning Score (NEWS): standardising the assessment of acute-illness severity in the NHS.* . Royal College of Physicians of London (2017). *National Early Warning Score (NEWS) 2* (December). .

46. For example, see Escher M, Ricou B, Nendaz M, et al. (2018). ICU physicians' and internists' survival predictions for patients evaluated for admission to the intensive care unit. *Annals of Intensive Care*, **8(108)**. https://doi.org/10.1186/s13613-018-0456-9 (accessed 11 June 2020).

47. Emanuel E, Persad G, Upshur R, et al. (2020). Fair allocation of scarce resources in the time of Covid-19. https://www.nejm.org/doi/full/10.1056/NEJMsb2005114 (accessed 11 June 2020).

48. Section 11 Coronavirus Act 2020 offers a clinical indemnity for claims in tort arising from the pandemic.

49. Gostin LO, Friedman EA, Wetter SA. (2020). Responding to Covid-19: how to navigate a public health emergency legally and ethically, *Hastings Center Report*, **50(2)**, 2. https://doi.org/10.1002/hast.1090 (accessed 11 June 2020).

50. The law was absolutely clear as to the requirement to involve the patient or (when they lacked capacity) those appropriately concerned with their welfare: see *R (Tracey) v Cambridge University Hospitals NHS Foundation Trust & Anor* [2014] EWCA Civ 33 and *Winspear v City Hospitals Sunderland NHS Foundation Trust* [2015] EWHC 3250 (QB).

51. See, for example, BBC News, 'Coronavirus: GP surgery apology over "do not resuscitate" form' (1 April 2020): https://www.bbc.co.uk/news/uk-wales-52117814 (accessed 11 June 2020). Requiring someone to complete their own DNACPR form was, in fact, legally impossible unless they were being asked to make advance decisions to refuse CPR, which would then require compliance with the statutory provisions of the Mental Capacity Act (MCA) 2005 (including that they be witnessed): see Section 25 MCA 2005.

52. See, too, the Department of Health & Social Care's 'Covid-19: Our action plan for adult social care' of 15 April 2020, stating that:

   It is unacceptable for advance care plans, including Do Not Attempt Resuscitation orders, to be applied in a blanket fashion to any group of people, and the CQC have been urgently contacting providers where this practice has been brought to their attention. Everyone at risk of losing mental capacity or nearing the end of their life should be offered the opportunity and supported, if they wish, to develop advance care planning that make their wishes clear, and to make arrangements, such as lasting power of attorney for health and social care decisions, to put their affairs in order. This must always be a personalised process. (Available at (https://assets.publishing. service.gov.uk/government/uploads/system/uploads/attachment_data/file/879639/ covid-19-adult-social-care-action-plan.pdf, accessed 11 June 2020).

53. See, for instance, the General Medical Council's guidance at https://www.gmc-uk.org/ ethical-guidance/ethical-hub/covid-19-questions-and-answers#Working-safely (accessed 11 June 2020), acknowledging that '[w]e do not expect doctors to leave patients without treatment, but we also don't expect them to provide care without regard to the risks to themselves or others. This pandemic is an unprecedented challenge in which clinicians are understandably balancing the imperative to provide care with their own fears.'

Index

Tables and figures are indicated by *t* and *f* following the page number

For the benefit of digital users, indexed terms that span two pages (e.g., 52–53) may, on occasion, appear on only one of those pages.